High-Powered Plyometrics

Second Edition

James Radcliffe

Robert C. Farentinos

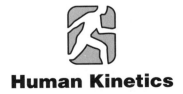

Human Kinetics

Library of Congress Cataloging-in-Publication Data

Radcliffe, James C. (James Christopher), 1958-
  High-powered plyometrics / James Radcliffe, Robert C. Farentinos. -- 2nd ed.
  pages cm
  Includes bibliographical references.
  1. Plyometrics. I. Farentinos, Robert C., 1941- II. Title.
  GV711.5.R326 2015
  613.7'1--dc23

2014043369

ISBN: 978-1-4504-9813-5 (print)

Acquisitions Editor: Justin Klug; **Developmental Editor:** Laura Pulliam; **Managing Editor:** Nicole O'Dell; **Associate Managing Editor:** B. Rego; **Copyeditor:** Patsy Fortney; **Proofreader:** Jan Feeney; **Graphic Designer:** Joe Buck; **Graphic Artist:** Tara Welsch; **Cover Designer:** Keith Blomberg; **Photographs (cover and interior):** © Human Kinetics; **Visual Production Assistant:** Joyce Brumfield; **Photo Production Manager:** Jason Allen; **Art Manager:** Kelly Hendren; **Associate Art Manager:** Alan L. Wilborn; **Printer:** United Graphics

We thank the University of Oregon in Eugene, Oregon, for assistance in providing the location for the photo shoot for this book.

Human Kinetics books are available at special discounts for bulk purchase. Special editions or book excerpts can also be created to specification. For details, contact the Special Sales Manager at Human Kinetics.

The video contents of this product are licensed for private home use and traditional, face-to-face classroom instruction only. For public performance licensing, please contact a sales representative at www.HumanKinetics.com/SalesRepresentatives.

Printed in the United States of America   10   9   8   7   6   5   4   3   2   1

The paper in this book is certified under a sustainable forestry program.

Human Kinetics
Website: www.HumanKinetics.com

United States: Human Kinetics
P.O. Box 5076
Champaign, IL 61825-5076
800-747-4457
e-mail: humank@hkusa.com

Canada: Human Kinetics
475 Devonshire Road Unit 100
Windsor, ON N8Y 2L5
800-465-7301 (in Canada only)
e-mail: info@hkcanada.com

Europe: Human Kinetics
107 Bradford Road
Stanningley
Leeds LS28 6AT, United Kingdom
+44 (0) 113 255 5665
e-mail: hk@hkeurope.com

Australia: Human Kinetics
57A Price Avenue
Lower Mitcham, South Australia 5062
08 8372 0999
e-mail: info@hkaustralia.com

New Zealand: Human Kinetics
P.O. Box 80
Torrens Park, South Australia 5062
0800 222 062
e-mail: info@hknewzealand.com

E6331

This book is dedicated to the most influential people a teacher and coach could have: parents Bill and Helen Radcliffe; Kathern Farentinos; mentors Mike Lopez Sr. and Clay Erro; and a wonderful colleague, partner, wife, and friend, Janice.

Contents

Part I   Plyometric Training

Get results using plyometrics
Apply athletic principles to plyometric training
Evaluate based on the various types of strength
Use the stretch–shortening concept

Activate power to create a successful training session
Warm up to properly prepare for work
Cool down to relax and recover

Maintain form and execution by following basic guidelines
Breathe to assist exercise execution
Train progressively to maximize skill
Use rest periods advantageously
Optimize training through the environment

Understand capabilities and limitations
Develop an effective program
Review power evaluation protocols

Part II Plyometric Exercises

Part III   Plyometric Programming

Drill Finder

Drill name	Drill #	Page #	Drill emphasis	Drill level	VOD included?
CHAPTER 5 UPPER-BODY POWER DEVELOPMENT					
Arm swing	10	74	Upper-body rhythm	Low	
Bench push-off	14	78	Upper-torso explosiveness	Moderate	
Catch and overhead throw	9	73	Upper-torso explosiveness	Shock	
Chest push	2	66	Upper-body explosiveness	Low	
Drop push-up	15	79	Upper-body explosiveness	Shock	▶
Heavy bag stroke	12	76	Upper-torso explosiveness	Moderate	▶
Heavy bag thrust	11	75	Upper-torso explosiveness	Moderate	▶
Kneeling two-arm overhead throw	6	70	Upper-body explosiveness	Moderate	
Medicine ball chest pass	1	65	Upper-body explosiveness	Low	▶
Multiple hops to overhead throw	19	83	Total body explosiveness	High	
Multiple hops to underhand toss	22	86	Total body explosiveness	High	▶
Push jerk	17	81	Total body explosiveness	Moderate	
Push press	16	80	Upper-torso explosiveness	Beginner	
Scoop toss	21	85	Total body explosiveness	Moderate	▶
Shovel toss	20	84	Upper-torso explosiveness	Beginner	
Sit-up throw	3	67	Upper-body explosiveness	Beginner	
Split jerk	18	82	Total body explosiveness	High	
Standing two-arm overhead throw	7	71	Total body explosiveness	High	
Stepping two-arm overhead throw	8	72	Total body explosiveness	High	
Supine one-arm overhead throw	4	68	Upper-body explosiveness	Low	
Supine two-arm overhead throw	5	69	Upper-body explosiveness	Low	
Wall push-off	13	77	Upper-body explosiveness	Low	▶
CHAPTER 6 CORE POWER DEVELOPMENT					
Balanced toss	31	96	Balance and stability	Low	▶
Bar kip-up	33	98	Hip whip	Moderate	

(continued)

Drill Finder (continued)

Drill name	Drill #	Page #	Drill emphasis	Drill level	VOD included?
CHAPTER 7 LOWER-BODY POWER DEVELOPMENT (CONTINUED)					
Extended skipping	55	124	Postural hip projection	High	●
Fast skipping	53	122	Postural hip projection	High	●
Galloping	52	121	Hip projection and reactivity	Low	●
Incline ricochet	79	148	Elasticity and reactivity	Low	
Incremental vertical hop	68	137	Postural control and reactivity	Low	●
Knee-tuck jump	41	110	Postural hip projection	Moderate	
Lateral bound	57	126	Postural hip projection	Moderate	●
Lateral stair bound	60	129	Postural hip projection	Moderate	●
Pogo	35	104	Hip projection and reactivity	Low	●
Power skipping	54	123	Postural hip projection	Moderate	●
Prancing	51	120	Hip projection and reactivity	Low	●
Quick leap	47	116	Postural hip projection	High	●
Rocket jump	38	107	Postural hip projection	Low	
Scissors jump	43	112	Postural hip projection	Moderate	●
Side hop	69	138	Postural control and reactivity	Low	●
Side hop-sprint	70	139	Postural control and reactivity	Low	
Single-leg diagonal hop	76	145	Postural control and reactivity	High	
Single-leg hop	74	143	Postural control and reactivity	High	
Single-leg lateral hop	77	146	Postural control and reactivity	High	
Single-leg pogo	72	141	Hip projection and reactivity	High	●
Single-leg slide kick	73	142	Postural control and reactivity	High	●
Single-leg speed hop	75	144	Postural control and reactivity	High	●
Single-leg stair bound	58	127	Postural hip projection	Moderate	●
Split jump	42	111	Postural hip projection	Low	●
Squat jump	36	105	Postural hip projection	Moderate	
Star jump	39	108	Postural hip projection	Moderate	
Stride jump	45	114	Postural hip projection	High	●
Stride jump crossover	46	115	Postural hip projection	High	●

Accessing the Online Video

This book includes access to online video that includes 53 clips demonstrating some of the most dynamic exercises discussed in the book. In the Drill Finder and throughout the book, exercises marked with this play button icon indicate where the content is enhanced by online video clips: ▶

Take the following steps to access the video. If you need help at any point in the process, you can contact us by clicking on the Technical Support link under Customer Service on the right side of the screen.

1. Visit www.HumanKinetics.com/HighPoweredPlyometrics.
2. Click on the **View online video** link next to the book cover.
3. You will be directed to the screen shown in figure 1. Click the **Sign In** link on the left or top of the page. If you do not have an account with Human Kinetics, you will be prompted to create one.

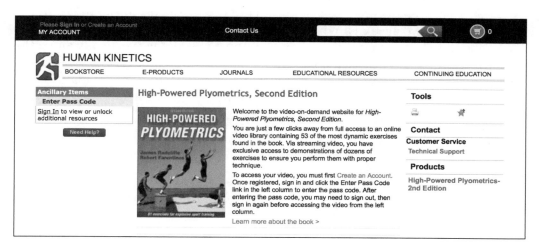

Figure 1

4. If the online video does not appear in the list on the left of the page, click the **Enter Pass Code** option in that list. Enter the pass code exactly as it is printed here, including all hyphens. Click the Submit button to unlock the online video. After you have entered this pass code the first time, you will never have to enter it again. For future visits, all you need to do is sign in to the book's website and follow the link that appears in the left menu.

Pass code for online video: RADCLIFFE-93RL4-OLV

5. Once you have signed into the site and entered the pass code, select **Online Video** from the list on the left side of the screen. You'll then see an Online Video page with information about the video, as shown in the screenshot in figure 2. You can go straight to the accompanying videos for each topic by clicking on the blue links at the bottom of the page.

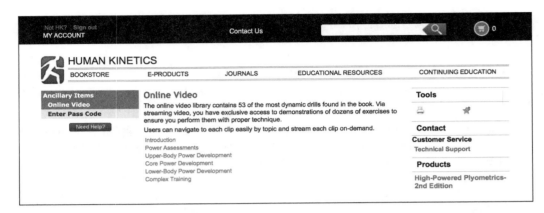

Figure 2

6. You are now able to view video for the topic you selected on the previous screen, as well as all others that accompany this product. Across the top of the page, you will see a set of buttons that correspond to the topics in the text that have accompanying video. Once you click on a topic, a player will appear. In the player, the clips for that topic will appear vertically along the right side. Select the video you would like to watch and view it in the main player window. You can use the buttons at the bottom of the main player window to view the video full screen, to turn captioning on and off, and to pause, fast-forward, or reverse the clip.

Foreword

Jim Radcliffe is almost always the smallest guy on the field or in the weight room. His passion, expertise, boundless energy, and conversational tone allow him to command a team of behemoths. The traditional strength and conditioning coach is nowhere to be found at the University of Oregon.

What are we doing on the field of play, the court, and certainly the track? How do we do it better—this includes smarter, safer, and more efficiently? Who is the person we are training? These are three questions that Coach Rad is constantly analyzing on a never-ending quest to answer.

Rad's style is impossible to demonstrate and communicate merely in book form. Two of the biggest challenges in teaching—demonstration and communication—are strengths rooted in his passion for personal and athletic excellence. He knows every student-athlete's goals, hopes, motivation, and perceived limitations. His one-on-one engagement allows him to push the athletes beyond their wildest dreams.

Coach Rad has led gold medalists, countless national champions, and hundreds of All-Americans. But that is not why he does it. He does it to see young men and women engage in a process of constant competitive excellence. These are lifelong traits that will stay with them well beyond any record, mark, or milestone.

While breaking things down into a manageable daily punch list, he challenges all of us as coaches to think big picture and long term. As you look at all the information and exercises in this book—the what—make it personal—the why. Take inventory of your motivation in doing certain things. Also, get to know your student-athletes and understand who they are. These measures will help all of you continually improve.

Coach Rad makes me a better coach and person every day. Whether you are a coach, athlete, physician, physical therapist, personal trainer, or weekend warrior, you will benefit from Coach Rad's passion as it comes through these pages.

Mark Helfrich
Head football coach
University of Oregon

Preface

Our main objective in presenting *High-Powered Plyometrics* is to offer the most systematic, comprehensive, and practical treatment of plyometrics available. This book provides concepts, practical information, training programs, and performance evaluation systems for this style of training.

During the last 30 years we have conducted an extensive program of plyometric training for fitness enthusiasts and high school and college athletes. Since the 1980s, intercollegiate and professional American football, baseball, and basketball players; world-class cross-country skiers; weightlifters; cyclists; track athletes; marathon and mountain runners; young athletes; and older fitness buffs have trained in plyometrics, among them several participants in the Olympic Games and World Championships. *High-Powered Plyometrics* is the result of extensive research and coaching, and especially of Jim Radcliffe's original and practical work during the past three and a half decades.

We wrote this book for coaches, athletes, sports medicine clinicians, and all who wish to know more about plyometrics and how to apply this dynamic training method to specific sports. We have expanded the original edition to include comprehensively defined training concepts, thorough teaching and training methodologies, and the latest research and practical considerations. A video and e-book complement this work.

We are deeply committed to plyometric training: we use it in our own workouts and in directing the training of others. We have extensively reviewed the professional literature in this area of training and present these findings along with our experiences. Many other books give good definitions of plyometric training and descriptions of how to set it up and perform certain exercises. *High-Powered Plyometrics,* however, is the first to provide a complete description of the principles behind the tasks of establishing training regimens and progressing optimally throughout specific exercise sequences for enhanced training and performance.

The term *plyometrics* was derived from the Greek word *pleythyein,* which means "to augment" or "to increase," and the shorter Greek words *plio* ("more") and *plyo* ("to move"). *Metrics* means "to measure" or "length." The spelling *pliometric* is also accepted in referring to eccentric contraction or muscle lengthening. The word *plyometrics* originally appeared in Russian sports literature in 1966 in the work of Zatsiorsky (Zanon 1989). American track and field coach Fred Wilt offered an explanation of the term in 1975, and many have followed. A few other terms have been associated with plyometrics as well, including *shock training, speed strength, bounce training,* and *elastic reactivity.*

Although we know some basic neuromuscular processes that underlie plyometrics, we must learn a great deal more before we fully understand how it works. Fortunately, research conducted by such sport scientists as Yuri Verkhoshansky, Carmelo Bosco, Paavo Komi, Gregory Wilson, Mel Siff, Maarten Bobbert, Warren Young, Vern Gambetta, and James Hay has paved the way for more and improved work with coaches and researchers such as Gary Winkler, Dean Benton, Ian King, Frans Bosch, Roald Klomp, Vladimir Zatsiorsky, Gabriele Wulf, Keith Davids,

William Ebben, and Peter Weyend. From a practical viewpoint, experience supports the significant value of plyometrics, even if, from a physiological perspective, explanations of why it works remain elusive.

A constant struggle to be practical yet scientifically accurate is common in the field of physical training. Every day we coaches and athletes try to do the things that will offer us the best results. We want to be efficient, and we would like the results to be reliable. This book lets coaches and athletes know the results they can expect from explosive training and provides clinical explanations for those results so they don't have to discover them themselves in the lab.

This text explains what is happening inside during plyometric training and why. We define plyometrics, present concepts, and describe the principles that explain how and why plyometrics works.

High-Powered Plyometrics explains how to know when you or your participants are ready to use the training methods, and how to get ready for them. The best training results come from methods that are used properly—not just explosively, but overall. The following pages explain the elements involved in preparing for training and performance, as well as equipment and basic exercises.

This book outlines the training elements and safety precautions needed for performing skillfully in sports, as well as the principles for executing plyometric exercises. Be sure to follow the guidelines for training safely.

Chapters 5, 6, and 7 constitute a field guide of training drills and drills as well as descriptions of basic plyometric movements related to the arms, trunk, and legs. In chapter 8 we explain the concepts of combining, or complexing, lifting and plyometric methods of training.

Finally, in chapters 9 and 10, we present a plan to continue with plyometric training at the most advanced levels. We also explain how to use progression, an aspect of plyometrics necessary at every workout level and in every athletic situation. In addition to discussing progression throughout the book, we describe each drill in the proper progressions. More than 200 photographs enhance the explanations of the concepts, movement execution, and sequential drills.

The objective is for you to better understand the concepts behind plyometric training and then use that knowledge to design and implement the most optimal application of plyometric work into training.

Note: If you use the metric system in your measurements, you can replace the number of yards with meters. Other units of measurements are converted.

Acknowledgments

We are grateful to many athletes and coaches who helped us with this book, especially Mike Lopez, who helped Jim Radcliffe with his initial endeavors in the plyometric area. We received valuable assistance from Clay Erro, Vern Gambetta, Rock Light, Gary Winkler, Frank Gagliano, Nick Symmonds, Vince Anderson, Mark Stream, Robert Johnson, Lou Osternig, Janice Lettunich Radcliffe, Pat Lombardi, Geoff Ginther, Dave Ziemba, Jeremy Pick, John Krazinski, Mark Dillon, Joel Favor, Art Tolhurst, Frans Bosch, Mark Rowland, the many athletes and coaches from the University of Oregon, and the wonderful Oregon Track Club athletes in Eugene. Also, thank you to Alexandra Davidson, Maggie Pietka, Tyler Pinkney, Chris Stubbs, and Nick Toreson. We have enjoyed the personal and professional associations with all concerned and truly hope we have returned the favor in some way.

Plyometric Training

Power Prerequisite for High-Level Performance

Plyometrics is a method of developing explosive power. It is also an important component of most athletic performances. As coaches and athletes have recognized the improvements plyometrics can bring to performance, they have integrated it into overall training programs in many sports and made it a significant factor in planning the scope of athletic development.

PLYOMETRICS AND POWER DEVELOPMENT

For some, reasons why plyometrics works may still be confusing, yet it is a fact that the training brings results. Yuri Verkhoshansky stated in the late 1960s that people could significantly improve their jumping and sprinting ability by performing progressive jumping exercises. The training and performances of athletes such as Olympic sprint champion Valeri Borzov helped to substantiate those statements. In the early 1980s, researchers Polhemus, Burkhardt, and others offered substantial evidence that combining plyometric training with a weight training program enhances physical development far beyond what can be achieved from weight training programs alone. Good combined programming was shown to enhance strength and speed and help athletes avoid injury. Since then, abundant research has shown that proper progressive training using these concepts not only fosters results in competition but also significantly decreases the number of catastrophic sport injuries, such as ACL tears and lower leg, foot, and ankle fractures (Hewitt et al. 1999).

People have probably always valued physical power, and, at least since the time of the ancient Greeks, athletes have sought methods for improving their speed and strength. Power, after all, is the combination of strength and speed, force times velocity. It is the application of force through a range of motion within a unit of time.

Power is essential in performing most sport skills, whether it's a tennis serve or a clean and jerk. Not surprisingly, then, specific exercises have long been designed to enhance quick, explosive movements. Yet only in the last few decades have programs been developed to systematically emphasize explosive–reactive power. Only more recently has explosive power training been refined.

In this age of technological advancements, we can analyze athletic performances with a great deal of instrumentation. GPS tracking and the ability to monitor athleticism in both sport contests and training have given more insight into the factors that separate high-level athletes and teams from the others. Elite teams, and a percentage of athletes on those teams, have a greater or more pronounced ability to burst and accelerate. This ability is a result of an optimal blend of force application and timing. Synchronization of these features, or the coordination of strong, fast multiple-movement skills, is the desired result of explosive power training.

PRINCIPLES OF PLYOMETRIC TRAINING

Certain principles of athletic development apply to plyometrics and the stretch–shortening cycle (SSC). Eccentric and concentric muscle actions usually occur simultaneously in combinations of muscle function known as the stretch–shortening cycle. The eccentric contraction stretches a muscle's length, and the concentric contraction shortens it. Most movements result from concentric actions preceded by eccentric countermovements. Defining the principles of the stretch–shortening cycle helps us understand not only what is occurring within training and performing, but also how to apply these principles. This understanding is useful in planning plyometric training.

Progressive Overload

Using the principle of progressive overload develops strength, power, and endurance. The relationship between increasing muscular strength and resistive overload using weights is well known. Repetitions of work at less than overload emphasize muscular endurance, not strength.

Because we are emphasizing power development, and because power is the function of force times distance over time, several overload methods can be used. However, rather than the traditional definition of power (strength times speed), the principle of overload exploits the true formula of power in planning training sessions.

A term often used instead of power training is *speed-strength*. It indicates the ability to reach maximal strength during the movement in a brief time—a ratio of maximal strength in a movement and the time to reach it (Matveyev 1977). Many sport scientists use the term to describe several correlating components of strength—primarily, absolute, explosive, starting, and reactive. At this point another view of power using a more definitive formula is appropriate, so let us take another view of power. In basic physics lectures on power, teachers always present the following formula, with these applications:

$$P = F \times d \, / \, t$$

F = application of force

d = application through the greatest distance

t = application in the least amount of time

Let's put into words what we are really after:

F = force application (i.e., strength and impulse)

d = distance transition (i.e., agility and coordination)

t = time reduction (i.e., speed and acceleration)

Few coaches would disagree with the statement that to apply more force (F), we must improve strength. Also, few would disagree that accelerated movements are required to reduce the time (t) factor. However, surprisingly, many coaches neglect to incorporate the formula's other equation—the agility and coordination needed for making appropriate distance transitions (d). The body's characteristics (e.g., size and shape) always set certain limitations, of course. Because athletes need all three components to make up the pie, in plyometric training they must plan to use overloads that will accomplish what they want in all these areas. The types of overloads available in plyometric training are shown in table 1.1.

In training the stretch–shortening cycle, resistive overloads usually take the form of rapidly stretching a limb or the entire body in an eccentric contraction, such as overcoming the increased g-forces as the result of falling from a height. To place a spatial overload on the stretch–shortening cycle, an athlete can increase the range, within a desired plane of movement, during the application of forces. Movement can also create the effects of overload through range of motion. The concept is to employ the stretch reflex within a specific range of motion. An example is an athlete performing a vertical jump from both feet without any approach. The application of force is upward, with all parts of the body summating forces in that direction. The athlete can apply the same summation of forces from a position in which the legs are split in the sagittal plane, increasing the overloads placed on the system and the degree of difficulty. Many exercises—although specific to particular athletic skills in terms of the movement plane of the limbs and the involvement of certain muscle groups—are executed in a spatially exaggerated manner; that is, limbs may move through much wider ranges of motion, even though the movement plane resembles that of the performance goal.

A temporal overload can be accomplished by executing the movement as rapidly and intensely as possible. The force the skeletal muscle produces depends on the speed of shortening or lengthening and the absolute length of the muscle at any instant in time. In eccentric exercise, force increases as the velocity of stretch increases. This is in contrast to concentric exercise, in which the force decreases as the speed of the contraction increases. One theory is that the faster the transition occurs from eccentric to concentric contraction, the greater the muscle tension produced and, potentially, the greater the muscle power produced (Komi 1973). Athletes can develop in this area by using decline pathways and springlike surfaces, as well as other variations.

Table 1.1   Types of Plyometric Overload

Resistive overload	Gravitational
	Inclination
	External
Spatial overload	Range
	Sagittal, transverse, frontal
Temporal overload	Operating rate
	Impulse

Dilemmas of Eccentric Exercise

Eccentric exercise has been shown to damage muscle cells and motor performance. However, various sport scientists (including Ebbeling and Clarkson 1990; Frid'en 1984; and Fritz and Stauber 1988) have found data suggesting that damaged connective tissue and muscle relates to important regeneration processes. The eccentric side of contraction also seems to cause increased intramuscular fluid pressure, a factor associated with delayed muscle soreness. An understanding of these concepts can help us better assess training, fatigue, overuse, and recovery.

Eccentric contractions cause more changes in certain muscle functions than do concentric contractions. These changes seem to be the result of trauma, initially in the mechanics. However, with time, chemical changes also occur. Greater forces during eccentric contractions, according to Curwin and Stanish (1984), also create greater stress on tendons.

The increased use of eccentric muscular exercise to augment performance and rehabilitation has generated questions about optimal and safe training loads. For practitioners, a great concern is the lack of consensus about appropriate volumes and intensities of eccentric loading exercises. Developments over the last 30 years, as a result of study and practical evaluation, have helped us greatly in dosage recommendations.

Eccentric muscle contraction deserves special consideration because it can absorb shock. Training using only eccentric actions eliminates the inhibitory actions allowing for improvement in muscle strength and function. This shows us a further need for examining the balance of eccentric and concentric muscle regimens and understanding the optimal use of eccentric and stretch–shortening cycle training methodologies (Stauber 1989).

Continued damage to myofibers and connective tissue and continued repair and adaptation are long-term training effects of repeated eccentric muscle actions, although recovery tends to be slow (i.e., 7 to 10 days). On the other hand, repeated bouts of eccentric exercise can produce adaptations before complete recovery and restoration. Repeated long-term eccentric tension reorganizes and recoordinates muscle fiber structures, resulting in better stretch ability and reduced mechanical damage. However, a fine line exists between the microtearing of muscle fiber that improves power and adaptation and that which is harmful. The difference lies in the work-to-rest ratio, such as using the higher-stress training only twice per week and attempting to get at least two days (48 to 72 hours) of active recovery between each training session of explosive and reactive nature. Examples of this are covered in the chapters that deal with planning.

A major way to address eccentric loading problems is to use force-reducing techniques such as prestretch exercises for the agonistic muscles, which help to maintain good mechanics and postural control. A premotion silent period, which involves stretching the agonist while reinforcing the dynamic forces to follow, seems to significantly reduce the forces in dynamic and ballistic movements (Aoki, Tsukahara, and Yabe 1989). Athletes can progress through rehabilitative phases using the same concepts. This coincides with the developments by Hewitt, Myer, and Ford (2005, 2006); Padua et al. (2009, 2011); and Onate et al. (2010) of protocols for injury assessments and progressive training to curb and even eliminate the incidence of ACL, ankle, foot, and soft tissue injuries.

For rehabilitation, this involves slow, controlled, eccentric movements developed to the point of being able to control much higher velocities with eccentric, contractile stopping abilities. In jumping in stretch–shortening cycle training, for instance, landing technique is the primary issue. How well a person lands dictates how well the person next takes off. By executing the proper prelanding posture and give with the landing impact, the impulsive reversal of motion becomes the ultimate feature of the training.

Specificity

Another tenet of athletic training central to plyometrics is the principle of specificity. In athletic training, specificity refers to neuromuscular and metabolic adaptations of particular types of overload. Exercise stress, such as strength training for certain muscle groups, induces specific strength adaptations in particular muscular areas. For example, increases in endurance can only be achieved by training for endurance. Specific exercises elicit specific adaptations, thus creating specific training effects (McArdle, Katch, and Katch 1981). To jump higher or farther, athletes must structure their practices around jumps in those parameters. For speed, they must work at operating rates that are specific to those objectives. Thus, the specific plyometric or stretch–shortening cycle training effect is a methodology to develop powerful muscular responses, which are achieved by using overloads not only at the resistive and temporal levels but also at the spatial levels. Achieving the desired training effect from the stretch–shortening cycle requires using particular levels of resistance, speed, and space (i.e., distance covered). Overloads in the areas of resistance, timing or speed, and space or distance are important considerations. Plyometrics involves controlled frequency, intensity, duration, and specificity of training.

Progress in this area of knowledge now hinges on two complications. First, several methods develop explosive or reactive power (or both). Some are general, others are more specific, and each has distinct characteristics. The second complication is that these methods have been researched, developed, practiced, and interpreted in several countries, languages, and structures of society.

This chapter explains the system of plyometric training by discussing how to do the following:

- Train rate of force development (RFD) and enhance not only maximal strength but also dynamic strength, or the type of forces developed at high velocities of movement.
- Use exercises requiring the utmost muscular effort against moderate resistance (dynamic effort).
- Employ specific exercises and methods that improve reversible muscle action, or stretch–shortening, which involves specific motor abilities (Zatsiorsky 1995).

JUDGING THE BEST QUALITIES IN POWER DEVELOPMENT

Sport scientists have raised some interesting questions about the amount of strength and stability necessary for successfully performing eccentric training, the effects of slower isotonic strength training on eccentric performance, and whether relationships exist between more ballistic (plyometric) training and isotonic training. Traditional weight training basically enhances muscular strength. Plyometric training, on the other hand, enhances muscular power. Greg Wilson (1993) and others suggested that athletes use dynamic weight training (a form of stretch–shortening cycle exercises that are externally loaded) to maximize mechanical output.

Continually evaluating the strength of a plyometric participant is important. Following are the forms of strength that should be evaluated:

- *Core strength*, which is discussed less often but may be the most basic and important of all
- *Absolute strength*, or the maximal level, which is measured regardless of body weight
- *Relative strength*, or maximal levels scaled to body weight, which is important in projecting the center of gravity away from, across, or over the ground
- *Dynamic strength,* which involves both eccentric and concentric contractions, with a degree of speed (used, for example, in squatting and single-response jumping movements where one repetition is performed at a time with a complete reset before the next rep)
- *Elastic strength,* which is speed involving the elastic and contractile components and reflex contractions (such as rebound, or multiple-response where reps are continuously repeated)

Core strength centers on the core of the body, defined here as the control over the muscles and joints of the trunk, or torso. It is responsible for all postural stability in movements in all planes and directions. Core strength is a component of all the other forms of strength. In handling any external loads or any speed of movement, core control influences the beginning, maintenance, and completion phases (see figure 1.1). We refer to this stabilizing effect of postural control often in the rest of this book. Everything we do in athletic performance begins from the core and radiates outward, and our training should do the same. So, rather than saving the concepts of improving the core until the end, we place it at the beginning of every training session.

Being able to demonstrate and assess strength qualities (e.g., starting, maximal, and explosive) makes an athlete more aware of the essential power qualities athletic performance demands. All forms of strength have a place in evaluation and should be prioritized according to the progressive objectives of the program. For example, an athlete may exhibit good or even great strength as tested in a barbell squat. He might be weak, however, in a vertical jump test, possibly indicating a lack of speed in the training load and poor dynamic strength. This becomes even more evident when he is unable to handle multiple-response movements, which indicates low levels of elastic strength. Schmidtbleicher (1992) suggested that different rates of force development are necessary for overcoming different loads, both internal and external, and that they also affect the movement time involved.

Traditional strength training methods have often fostered the belief that maximal strength methods increase maximal strength and speed strength methods develop power. This belief often confuses people about the aim and

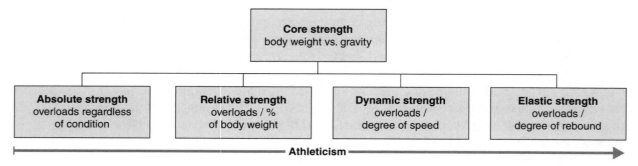

Figure 1.1 Hierarchy of physical adaptation to progressive gravitational stress.

content of training methods. Schmidtbleicher (1992) pointed out that an increase in maximal strength is always connected with an improvement in relative strength and therefore with an improvement in power capabilities. Once maximal strength capabilities have been enhanced, the objective of developing power and velocity of movement must be attended to; the rate of force development (RFD) must become the primary training objective. In sport, often the time available for force development is short, requiring RFD to take priority over maximal strength. An athlete who can squat or pull an extremely heavy load yet needs several seconds to do so is better served by lifting a slightly lighter load faster—that is, with a higher force rate. Weyend and colleagues (2000) referred to this as mass-specific strength, and they asserted that producing great force rapidly is more desirable than producing a greater force slowly.

Dynamic strength, or the forces developed in high-velocity movements such as sprinting, jumping, and high-speed changes of direction, is the next priority. This segment of training is also where accurate assessments can be of service, which is covered in chapter 4. Finally, the proverbial icing on the cake must be the development and improvement of the stretch–shortening cycle, or as Zatsiorsky (1995) suggested, reversible muscle action. When muscles shorten immediately after stretching, they can produce greater mechanical power with less metabolic energy cost.

At the foundation of the comprehensive training in this book are a few principles whose value is clear from experience. One is using to full advantage the power from eccentric contractions. A second is the advantage gained from exploiting the stretch–shortening cycle and the explosive power available from the elastic components of muscle. A third is adapting to plyometric programs the training principles of progressive overload and specificity, which we discussed earlier in this chapter.

When analyzing and applying training that uses the stretch–shortening cycle model, we must remember that athletic skills are never merely the sum of such factors as strength, velocity, loading, and stretch. Performance of any movement pattern, plyometric or otherwise, is holistic. It involves an integration of all such factors. During the development of power, many mechanisms drive and coordinate the skeletal musculature. Enhancing the muscular control and reactive power associated with stretch–shortening cycle exercise relates to changes in complex neuromuscular structure and sensorimotor pathways.

When muscles shorten immediately after a stretch, force and subsequent power output increases while the amount of energy expended decreases; thus, greater power uses less metabolic energy. The key factor lies in the transition from lengthening to shortening, known for our purposes as the coupling moment. It is at this coupling moment that force is developed, not in eccentric or concentric but rather in more isometric conditions. Coupling time, which has a very important impact on the optimization of plyometric work, is explained in detail in later chapters.

Before we discuss the phases of the stretch–shortening cycle, let's first take a look at how it works. Various terms have been suggested to describe phases of the stretch–shortening cycle, which includes the stretch or eccentric phase, the brief period between, and the shortening, or concentric, phase. Basically, the cycle combines an eccentric contraction, in which the involved muscles undergo tension through lengthening or stretching (negative work), and a concentric contraction, in which the muscles shorten (positive work). Figure 1.2 shows the cycle in its clinical form of muscle function and as it appears in its natural form. Komi (1984)

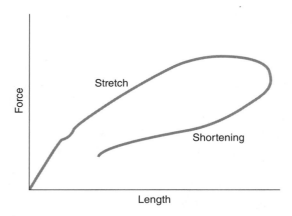

Figure 1.2   Clinical viewpoint of the stretch–shortening cycle.

described this effect of overcoming inertia as pushing a box end over end versus initial pushing of a wheel.

Loading and the Stretch Response

A muscle's initial length when stimulated influences the magnitude of its contractile responses. Applying force against a muscle, or loading, causes a reaction to the stress. When this load is applied, the amount of deformation (called strain) is the change that occurs in dimension. A liquid within the muscle resists these deformations during stretching and shortening; this resistance to flow is known as viscosity. It is because of the viscosity that muscles must move in the direction opposite the desired force application (this is called prestretch). The property of muscle tissue that enables greater muscular tension is known as the stretch response. Not to be confused with the stretch reflex (a basic neural mechanism to maintain active muscle tonus using impulses discharged from muscle spindles), the stretch response involves parallel muscle fibers·exerting maximal tension at stretch lengths slightly greater than resting length.

The concept of the prestretch has been confusing for many coaches and practitioners; many correlate it with muscle length or strength enhancement. To alleviate some of the confusion, we explain it as Frans Bosch (2005), Gary Winkler (2009), and others suggest, as pretension and the avoidance of slack in the systematic execution of contractions. Pretension is preparing for contact, or impact, by contracting, or stiffening, and thereby tensing the components of muscle, joint, and tendon. This synchronization, or coordination, of cocontractions reduces slack and optimizes the efficiency of contact. Truly improving the elastic–reactive potential of the neuromuscular system requires synchronizing the tendons, ligaments, and fascia (intramuscular), and then the muscles (intermuscular).

Elasticity

Muscle strength is the maximal force or tension that a muscle can generate. This is the force or tension a muscle group can exert against a resistance in one maximal effort. An important component accompanying strength is the muscle's elasticity (its ability to lengthen and increase in tension), which resides in the contractile elements of skeletal muscle. Naturally, there are limits to these abilities.

The range of elasticity, or strain, is directly proportionate to the ability of the tissue to resist forces and return to its original shape upon releasing a load. This is the elastic property that plyometric training addresses. Elasticity lends the ability to use the strain, or tension, to return to, or react, in the original direction with greater force, greater efficiency, or both. It is the basis for resilience, or the ability to absorb energy within the elastic range of the muscle. When a load is removed and the tissue returns to its original shape, resilience releases energy.

Studying elasticity has led to the concept of stored elastic energy, which is the recoverable energy the viscoelastic tissue deformation generates in the eccentric phase of the movement. This energy is available for reuse in the following concentric phase of muscle activity. Elastic energy has also been explained as mechanical energy that the muscle does not dissipate as heat but rather absorbs and stores for reuse during its subsequent active shortening cycle.

The basis of both the voluntary and involuntary motor processes involved in the stretch–shortening cycle is the so-called stretch reflex, which is also called the muscle spindle reflex or myotatic reflex. This spindle apparatus and the stretch reflex are vital components of the nervous system's overall control of body movement. When executing most movement skills, the muscles receive some type of load. The rapid stretching (loading) of these muscles activates this myotatic reflex, which sends a strong stimulus through the spinal cord to the muscles. This stimulus causes them to contract powerfully.

Springlike elements located in series (series elastic component, or SEC) or parallel (parallel elastic component, or PEC) to the myofilament of skeletal muscle are tension activated (Hill 1950). Muscles store elastic energy during eccentric work and recover it during concentric work. If amortization is slow, muscles dissipate elastic energy, usually as heat (Cavagna 1977). Elasticity is enhanced when the pretension and exchange duration is minimal (Komi 1973). Researchers believe the rate of stretch to be more important than its length or magnitude. The desire is for quick prestretch movements over longer, slower ones (Bosco and Komi 1979; Cavagna 1977). The rate of the stretch (and pretension) is more important than the magnitude (or length) of the stretch.

At this point the concept of slack must be addressed. As mentioned previously, and will be explained again in further chapters, tension is more important than stretch in plyometric training. A good deal of research has shown that a concentric contraction must occur to bring a muscle to a certain length, stretch the elastic components, and therefore obtain the right level of tension. The time it takes for this contraction to achieve a workable length is called rise latency. Rise latency adversely affects muscles needing to explode and negotiate the contact point quickly and efficiently. What is needed is a counteractive force moment. Sufficient tension must be present in the muscle before external forces are encountered (pretension, or rigidity). This reactive movement involves (1) pretensing the muscle (spring-loading), (2) landing and further stretching the series elastic components (SEC) and the antagonistic moment on the contractile elements (CE), which (3) reach maximal force for another concentric contraction.

As with optimal running, in which ground contact is short as a result of upright posture, SEC elasticity and CE rigidity create a rapid, forceful reactivity, or effortless bounce. As explained in detail in chapters 2 and 7 on technique, a neutral position of the ankle to create a well-timed plantarflexion just prior to ground contact prepares the musculature for impact, combined with a reduction in slack time at contact.

Perhaps the most accurate term to describe the time from the eccentric, or stretch, portion of the cycle through switching to the concentric, or shortened, portion is *elastic reactivity,* a concept that Gambetta described in 1986. What is important in elastic reactivity is the impulse, or the force that starts a body into motion, and the motion this force produces. Greater impulse relates to better efficiency. When greater stretches precede positive work, increased mechanical efficiency results. Called potentiation (see Komi 1986), the mechanics explain the synergistically augmented energy levels and heightened effectiveness.

Muscle Contractions

The human body is continually subject to external forces and impacts, against which muscles contract. Their contractions (or actions, a term preferred by some physiologists) are both negative (eccentric) and positive (concentric). In eccentric contractions, the muscles undergo tension and lengthen, or stretch (called negative work); in concentric contractions, they undergo tension and shorten (called positive work). Any external force a muscle experiences that is greater than its internal tension force allows it to lengthen in an eccentric contraction. This type of contraction enables the muscle to brake skeletal movements—in other words, to decelerate. An eccentric contraction allows a muscle to sustain greater tension than it can develop in an isometric position. Because the load applied to the muscle causes it to work by lengthening, it is called negative work (in contrast to the positive work done in concentric contraction to overcome resistance). That is, when muscles contract eccentrically, they lengthen as they simultaneously produce force. The external load is greater than the internal muscular force it can apply. Basically, every movement in the direction of gravity is under the control of an eccentric contraction.

What is significant here is that the energy cost of negative work is less than that of positive work. The body requires less motor unit activation and consumes less oxygen in eccentric contractions than it does in concentric contractions. Thus, the relationship between the input and output of energy differs between the two—eccentric exercise is more mechanically efficient than concentric exercise.

In eccentric actions performed at moderate to high speeds, the muscles call on fast-twitch muscle fiber units to work; they are thus preferentially recruited. They have higher firing frequencies and are larger fibers and produce more force per motor unit than other muscle fiber types do. Force production is greater during eccentric contraction than during concentric contractions because the body generates a higher tension at the point of the muscle's insertion. The tendon at insertion receives larger loads during eccentric exercise than it does during concentric exercise.

In summary, because of chemical, mechanical, and neurological factors that influence the force and stiffness of the contracting muscle (see Komi 1973), eccentric lengthening (before rapid concentric shortening) produces the greatest force and power capabilities in skeletal muscle. It is therefore the central type of contraction in plyometrics.

Proprioception and Potentiation

Perceptions of motion are transmitted from the muscle to the spinal cord to the brain and back to the muscle, regulating body movement via musculoskeletal sensory organs, interpretation by the central nervous system, motor unit recruitment, and muscle stiffness.

Training with a prestretch (and what we now understand to be pretensing) and activating neuromuscular components improves the efficiency of neural actions and muscular performance (Bosch and Klomp 2005; Schmidtbleicher 1992). Exercises that use the stretch–shortening cycle, or plyometrics, stimulate changes in the neuromuscular system, thereby enhancing the ability of the muscle groups to respond quickly and powerfully to slight and rapid changes in muscle length. An important feature is that the exercises condition the neuromuscular system to allow faster and more powerful changes of direction.

An increasing amount of research is being performed in the area of evaluation and risk factors as a result of improper landing mechanics and their effect on injuries such as ACL tears and stress fractures in the lower leg and foot. Padua and colleagues (2009) stated that movement patterns are important and modifiable factors that may influence the risk of lower-extremity injuries. Establishing the proper proprioceptive and potentiated landing patterns has been shown to be an effective way not only to improve performance but also to decrease the chances for the aforementioned injuries. As mentioned earlier and further emphasized throughout the book, using exercise progressions to establish proper landing mechanics establishes the movement and motor patterning that enhance safety and performance.

Plyometric exercises that isolate sections of the body for training can be formulated. They involve an array of jumps, bounds, and hops; flexions, extensions, and trunk rotations; and tossing, throwing, and passing. Descriptions and definitions of these moves are provided in chapters 5 through 7, and these are merely some of the many movements possible for exploiting the stretch–shortening cycle.

Amortization

As a general term, amortization is the gradual extinction, extinguishing, or deadening of something; in relation to the stretch–shortening cycle, it refers to the time that elapses from the beginning of the eccentric contraction phase to the beginning of the concentric contraction phase (see figure 1.3).

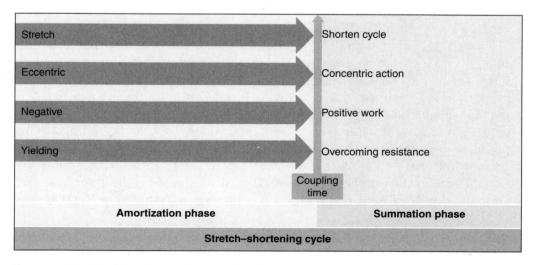

Figure 1.3   Terminology of amortization.

Minimizing the time lapse between eccentric and concentric contraction is extremely important for improving movement efficiency. Two periods of delay exist. One is between the signal from the brain for muscle contraction and the onset of muscle activity, and the other is between the appearance of muscle electric activity and the development of tension in the muscle, the electromechanical delay (EMD). The EMD is shorter in eccentric contractions than in concentric ones. This shortened response time underscores the importance of producing the greatest force in the least amount of time. The stretch–shortening mechanism enhances force production as a result of contributions from the series elastic component (SEC) during stretching. Eccentric efficiency, in other words, is improved by using the stored elastic energy of the SEC.

DETERMINING FACTORS IN THE STRETCH–SHORTENING CYCLE

Evaluating the factors involved with stretch–shortening cycle exercises determines timing, volumes, and intensities. King (1993) outlined these factors:

- Rate of eccentric action, known to many as the amortization phase (the stretch)
- Rate of concentric action, the recoil, or summation phase (shortening)
- Delay between the cessation of eccentric muscle action and onset of concentric muscle action, also known as coupling time
- Amount, if any, of the external load involved

These elements take only approximately half a second to occur, yet they can change the scope of the training form (see figure 1.4, a-d). We often need to distinguish a rapid continuous stretch–shortening cycle movement, or intensive elastic and reactive method, from those of a speed-strength orientation (loaded and not as elastic or reactive) or, furthermore, from a shock methodology. Schmidtbleicher (1992) considered these differences to be long or short stretch–shortening cycles—those greater or less than 250 milliseconds. In figure 1.4 the down portion indicates the amount of stretch; the up section shows the shortening and the combination of the two and the delay, if any, between them (coupling). These are all in the contact portions of the chart. Notice the differences in time necessary for executing minimal contact time and maximal flight.

Siff and Verkhoshansky (1996) suggested that if the coupling time is longer than about 0.15 second in exercises that require high impact, intensity, or rate of force, the action is not considered classical shock method plyometrics, such as depth jumping. For our purposes, knowing how to measure these times is not as important as understanding the differences individual exercises make, especially when incorporating greater movement magnitudes, such as bounding versus hopping, or greater gravitational overloads, such as dropping from greater heights or using additional weight on the body.

Coaches can evaluate performance based on an awareness of the ground contact or coupling time an athlete displays. The load can be determined by the response via ground contact time.

A theoretical understanding and observation of posture, balance, stability, and flexibility are required to determine what is occurring during fast movements. Because a great deal of stretch–shortening cycle improvement depends on the rate

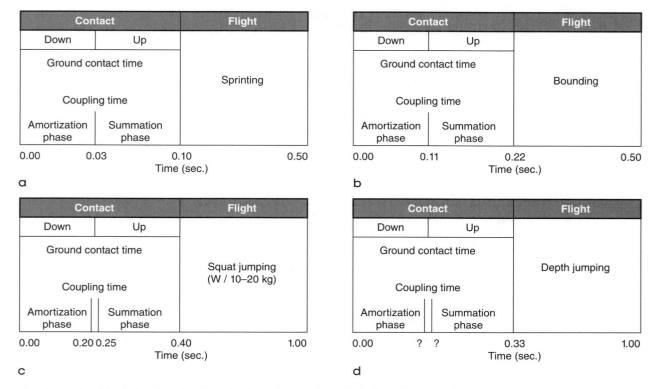

Figure 1.4 Stretch–shortening factors based on training form: *(a)* sprinting, *(b)* bounding, *(c)* squat jumping, and *(d)* depth jumping.

of force development and the development of neuromuscular coordination, coaches need to think carefully about the style, progressive application, and specificity of plyometric exercises. For example, training using squat jumps with 15 to 20 kilograms (33 to 44 lb) of external weight (e.g., a sandbag or weight vest) is useful in certain phases and progressive times of training, as is bounding for certain prolonged distances. However, for sprinters, this type of stretch–shortening cycle methodology doesn't address their need for quicker, more impulsive repetitions of higher quality the way lower-repetition bounding, hopping, or well-performed shock training does.

Repetitions of duration, external weight, and drops from height are best avoided until an athlete is far up the skill proficiency scale. Repetitions that sacrifice quality for quantity are also best avoided. However, the stretch–shortening cycle can be used throughout a continuum of exercise and load factors. An evaluation of the goals of each training phase and the sessions within those phases will indicate where (along the continuum) the majority of stretch–shortening cycle volume can fall. Examples of this evaluation system are in chapter 4 (the continuum of stress and complexity).

To continue our discussion of the concept of slack and using biological and biomechanical systems to better negotiate the ground, we expand on the aspects of more rigid segmenting of the body via cocontractions. First, an erect body posture is required. For our purposes, erectness does not always mean completely perpendicular to the ground; rather, it is the straight, rigid stiffness of the segments in relation to enhanced vertical contact points. This is covered in more detail in further chapters. A short coupling time is also necessary for reducing and enhancing the time spent on the ground. Finally, pretension prior to ground contact (stiffness) is needed, as is favoring the vertical aspects of landing and loading over the horizontal.

If the body were a stick figure, the goal would be to have the fewest angles, or breaks, in the figure. Some high jump coaches use a sawed-off crossbar as an example of this concept. They bounce the rod on its end to demonstrate the stiff bar's propulsion off the ground, lack of deformation at contact, and immediate rise up and over the high jump crossbar. In the animal world this stiffness concept is widely seen in the jumping and bouncing of deer and gazelle, also known as stotting (i.e., bounding with a stiff-legged gait). The more breaks or deformations in the segments, the greater the give on ground contact. Conversely, without some bend in the joints that enable the stretch–shortening cycle to work, where would the spring-loading occur?

An understanding of the intermuscular coordination of isometrically contracting the joints in preparation for contact and subsequent takeoff is important. The process of postural control and synchronized stiffening, thereby loading the spring of the activated musculature, enhances the ability to negotiate the contact surface. This concept has application for more than just the foot and the ground, as explained in later chapters.

We like to refer to the preceding concepts as negotiating contacts more like a superball than like a tomato. A tomato bounces but not for long or without a great deal of deformation, whereas a superball maintains its elasticity and rigidity. The concepts in this chapter help to optimize these qualities.

Athletic Power Activation Process

Chapter 1 addressed the concepts and qualities that factor into powerful performance. The biological and biomechanical aspects now become working parts of a process for activating athletic power. The biological aspect involves the neuromuscular system and other systems that boost power activation. Muscular contractions, responses, and contractile qualities, as well as neural pathways, all play parts in movement coordination.

GENERAL CONCEPTS OF POWER TRAINING

In training with plyometric exercises, as in other forms of stretch–shortening cycle or athletic training, it is important to follow guidelines to ensure safety as well as proper and effective performance. This chapter focuses on basic aspects of training that are the keys to good technique. The following six basic elements make up a good training session:

1. *Warm-up*: General (hip mobility walking exercises, lunging, crawling), core (abdominal, low back), and specific (technique work, skipping, accelerating)
2. *Dynamic work*: Explosive movements (e.g., snatches, jumps, throws, starts)
3. *Strength work*: Heavy multiple-joint movements (e.g., squats, jerks, loaded sprints)
4. *Isolated work*: Lying or seated movements (e.g., bench work, pulleys)
5. *Mobility work*: Fluid, full-body movements (e.g., agilities, stretching, recovery strides)
6. *Cool-down*: Stretching, movement flexibility work (or mobility), manual massage therapies, and cold immersion activities

Warm-Up

Because plyometric exercises emphasize posture, balance, flexibility, stability, and mobility, an adequate warm-up should precede all exercises. Preparatory warm-up routines should include progressive and aggressive dynamic movements that increase the temperature, viscosity, blood flow, and metabolism of the musculature, all of which ensure that the musculoskeletal system is activated and prepared. Aggressively performing dynamic and specific warm-up routines ensures optimal preparation for quality work.

As Warren Young (2002) and others suggested, the dynamic warm-up is a rehearsal for a specific skill; performed properly, it increases the proprioceptive efficiency of the neural pathways involved with each movement, activates specific motor units, and prepares the body skillwise both biomechanically and psychologically. In response to the debate over passive flexibility versus dynamic mobility, many studies in the past several years have shown that the passive approach, thought to be best for injury prevention, has not shown a higher correlation with injury prevention than the dynamic approach, although it does show performance decrements (Cramer 2005; Shrier 2004).

Following are sample exercises that make up a general warm-up with specific skill rehearsal (hip mobility walking exercises, lunging, and crawling). This is followed by technical form work that progresses from walking to skipping and running tempos (forward, lateral, and backward), core work (posture, balance, stability, mobility), specific lifting warm-up skills (using a light bar or stick in pulling, squatting, and pushing movements).

General

Walk—Knee to chest, marching

Lunge—Forward, side to side, and backward

Crawl—Hands and heels on the ground

Skip—Stepping and hopping with simulated sprinting mechanics

Shuffle—Side-to-side glide without crossing the feet

Carioca—Grapevine movement of step, step behind, step, step in front, twisting the hips

Backward movement—Lead with the feet and reach back trying to gain as much ground with each stride

Flexibility

Neck rotation

Shoulder roll

Shoulder rotation

Trunk twist

Hip rotation

Knee roll

Ankle rotation

Leg swing

Intramuscular Rehearsal

Forward

Mach drill—Walk, skip, and run routines of acceleration (A) and speed mechanics (B)

Fast skip—Emphasizing push and dynamic leg and hip mechanics

Slide kick—Emphasizing high heel recovery upward rather than backward

Rhythm and cadence—Interval combinations of sprint and stride mechanics with one leg

Fast leg cadence—Continuous sprint and stride combinations one leg at a time

Lateral

Shuffle—Side-to-side step routine using long, efficient strides and a low hip posture

Lateral skip—Side-to-side step-hop routine using a low hip posture

Backward

Backward run—Mimicking a forward running posture while moving backward

Backpedal—Maintaining a low hip posture, taking short strides that remain underneath the torso while moving backward

Backward skip—Backpedal posture with a step-hop foot cadence

Backward shuffle—Shuffle steps back with pivots continuously while facing forward

Backward kick-slide—Galloping effect of a back leg kick and reach with a foreleg push

Pulling

Good morning

Stiff-leg deadlift

Pushing

Behind-the-neck press

Military press

Alternating press

Squatting

Overhead squat

Overhead lunge

45-degree, or side, lunge

The exercises in a warm-up prepare the body to sprint, jump, cut, and move. They mobilize and technically prepare the system for fast and explosive performance. They also progress from walk to sprint tempo, yet always have an aggressive and dynamic quality. So, why these exercises and not jogging, butt kicks, stationary cycling, and so on? Those exercises, which tend to address the knee joint, not the hips, foster poor running and jumping form. Moreover, they are usually performed at tempos and using volumes of repetitions that are hard to reverse and relearn in the proper technique segment. Preparing for explosive movement should involve both proper technique and the correct execution rate. These are the questions to ask: What warm-up exercises foster better movement mechanics? What exercises foster poor movement mechanics?

After the warm-up, core warmth must be maintained, which is not determined by external sweating or the warmth of the environment. Here's a good example: An athlete spends the proper amount of time warming up and then performs a lying-down or seated exercise as her first activity (e.g., bench press). After 10 to 15 minutes of this, she decides to do a squatting, pulling, or jumping exercise. She still feels warm and is perspiring, but her body has been lying down all that time, even as she was pushing or moving with intensity. This is an example of poor session design because, although the athlete feels warm, her core muscular condition went down. Even though she got back to pulling and squatting and still felt warm, this condition is more external than internal (spinal and pelvic). The recommended workout segments that follow provide a good example of session management with an emphasis on explosive power.

Main Training Session

The main training session must be short but intense. Its design must ensure timely execution to preserve the warmth of the musculoskeletal systems and maintain their energy.

Off-season workout sessions should be approximately one hour long and include a warm-up and cool-down. Depending on the set, repetition, and rest methodology of some lifting situations, some workouts may last 15 or 25 minutes longer. Likewise, conditioning sessions that require maximal rest between plyometric and speed and agility sets may exceed an hour. However, for optimal development, these situations should not occur on a regular basis.

The optimal workout should include an efficient and complete warm-up, maintain core warmth throughout the workout, and include an adequate cool-down and recovery session to prepare for the next workout.

In relation to the concepts of optimal power performance training, the following points are key factors in the preparation, performance, and the follow-up of training practices.

- The warm-up should be followed by the portion of the training that is most dynamic and explosive (i.e., Olympic lifts, jumps, throws, starts, and accelerations).
- The heaviest or most strenuous portion of the workout should follow the fast and explosive portion (e.g., squatting, lunging, sled towing, sandpit).
- The third or close-to-final portion of the workout should involve smaller isolated movements such as bodybuilding, rehabilitative therapeutic exercises, and lying or sitting exercises (e.g., bench or incline lifts; machine exercises; shoulder, elbow, wrist, hip, knee, and ankle isolation exercises).
- The workout should always finish with mobility work—fluid full-body movements that provide intrinsic recovery as well as optimal movement efficiency training (e.g., agilities, barefoot striding and directional work, backward running and striding, stretching, rolling).

Table 2.1 is a sample time line of normal workout sessions, one in a weight room and the other in a conditioning field.

Table 2.1 Sample Time Line for Weight Room and Field Workouts

Time	Weight room	Conditioning field
:00	Dynamic warm-up	Dynamic warm-up
:05	Core or pillar work	Hip or mobility work
:12	Technical lift warm-up	Technical form movements
:20	Developmental lifts	Plyometrics and sprint training
:45	Mobility or isolated lifts	Agility or mobility exercises
:55	Cool-down or stretch	Cool-down stride and stretch

Cool-Down

A cool-down, the final portion of the workout session, should be performed in a relaxed yet productive and efficient manner. Immediately following the workout, the athlete should perform activities that provide adequate recovery and restoration to ensure continued quality training.

Increased blood flow throughout the system is a high priority during the cool-down. This can be achieved with external manipulation or internal movement activation. The following sections describe activities that can be included in a cool-down.

Sprint Preparation Work

Specific work involved in the development of sprint performance was mentioned in the warm-up section. The A and B series of sprint preparation, otherwise known as Mach drills, are named after Gerard Mach, the Polish and then Canadian sprint coach who invented sequences of specific sprint strengthening exercises. His purpose behind the evolution of the exercises was to continue muscular development via a rhythmic coordination of movement skills, each emphasizing a specific component of the proper powerful sprinting process. Polish winters and lack of adequate sprinting space became the catalyst for such drill work to take place, often in hallways and small gymnasiums.

Controversy exists regarding the use of the A and B series for sprint training. This is as it should be, because the drills are often used for a variety of technique work, warm-up routines, and form running. The main purpose of the drills is to use sprint muscles without having to do repeated full-out sprints. They are not form and technique drills by design. Athletes can improve acceleration technique sooner and more consistently by using resistance such as hills and sleds. The use of Bs for technique work can often bog down the learning curve rather than assist it. Our best use of these drills is for training sprinting more often. One of our best uses is as rehabilitation and recovery training from injuries to the hamstring, hip flexor, groin, and low back, because a good portion of these injuries result from hip immobility, a lack of postural integrity, and using the pendulum-at-the-knee technique instead of the piston-at-the-hip technique. Poor running postures and overstriding can be eliminated with the use of these progressions.

Stretching

The age-old failsafe for cool-downs is stretching, which can take multiple forms that provide various advantages.

- *Passive stretching*—the patient, relaxed hold of stretched muscle groups for 30 seconds or longer—is still practiced during warm-ups. However, research has shown it to be much more beneficial to overall performance and improvement at the conclusion of workouts, during the cool-down.
- *Active isolated stretching* involves using a strap, rope, or partner to stretch targeted muscles and then extending the stretch range by contracting and relaxing the antagonistic muscles of those under the stretch.
- *PNF, or contract–relax stretching*, involves a partner who helps hold targeted muscles in stretch as in passive stretching. After several seconds the partner provides light resistance while the athlete contracts the targeted (agonist) muscle groups to move the area back to the normal (unstretched) position. Once completed, the stretch is resumed with a greater range and ease of motion. This can be repeated two or three times, always ending with the relaxed portion of the stretch, rather than the contracted portion.

Movement Flexibility and Mobility

Movement flexibility work, or mobility work, also assists in posttraining recovery. Following are some forms:

- *Barefoot movement exercises*—Because there are more bones, joints, and small muscles in the feet and ankles, movements forward, backward, and in a variety of directions at moderate intensities aid in recovery and improved developmental capacity. Proper foot and ankle positioning for ground preparation is easier when the toes are exposed. The bottom of the foot is developed and massaged simultaneously, and when performed on grass or dirt, some researchers suggest the existence of a therapeutic effect known as earthing.
- *Crawling and climbing*—As when used in the warm-up, crawling and climbing are simple, quick, and low-intensity activities that open and close, thereby mobilizing, the muscles that surround the hips (low back, flexors, extensors, hamstrings, adductors and abductors, and quads).
- *Backward running*—Backward running helps establish proper upper-body running mechanics. It opens up the hip flexors after intense sprinting, bounding, and hopping, and it loosens up the hamstrings.

Cold Immersion

Another increasingly popular form of recovery is cold immersion, which comes in the following forms:

- Hot and cold contrast
- Ice baths
- Cool tub mobility movements
- Deep freeze chambers

Smarter Strength Training

In any type of improvement process, the underlying question is always How do we get better? For our purposes, the answer is simply to train smarter (Erro 1995). The ethos for most truly dedicated types is to work hard. Hard work is only good, however, if the work is smart. Hard work for hard work's sake is just work (e.g., *I am perspiring and breathing hard, and I'm sore and tired, so the work must be productive*).

As mentioned briefly in the warm-up section, some work is just hard work, yet not performance based. In this case, the athlete is practicing failure, performing reps until all technique, rate of operation, and performance quality has disappeared. This happens in explosive power training all the time. Plyometric "power hours" in an aerobics class and timed circuits of plyometric and explosive lifting movements that push the repetitions to poor performance levels, just for the sake of a good, hard workout, are examples.

As discussed in later chapters, quality should always come before quantity in plyometric training. Often, it is not just excessive quantity that leads to practicing failure; it is failing to remember the concepts of performance. Training smarter means having a good understanding of the concepts in this and the previous chapter. Understanding coupling time and better ground negotiation aids in the ability to plan, program, and execute successful training.

The two most common examples of hard versus smart training involve hurdle hopping and jumping and bounding. Hurdle hopping is a very popular plyometric training exercise. As long as the athlete can clear the hurdle with all of the elements of ground negotiation (upright postural control, short coupling and contact times, pretension, and vertical, pistonlike landings), then training can be successful. Coaches often believe that raising the hurdles makes for a better (harder) workout. However, the athlete may be working so hard to clear the hurdle that the proper elements of ground negotiation have flown out the window. In the case of jumping, bounding, and especially depth jumping with extra load (e.g., increased drop height, bungees, weight vests), again the concept has some merit because there is a strength component to having to handle such loads upon landing. The problem is that this type of strength development has negative ramifications not only to overall performance but also to the athlete's health. The longer the athlete is on the ground, the more bad things can happen.

Remember from chapter 1 the superball versus tomato analogy. Proper ground negotiation can be as easy to determine as whether the athlete is on and off the ground more like a superball or more like a tomato. A dropped tomato bounces, but not very well and with a great deal of deformation. Increasing the height of the drop or adding extra load to the tomato only leads to less bounce and greater deformation until eventually . . . splat! As long as the athlete's ground negotiation is superball-like, the training can be good quality work. Once tomato-ness is observed, the athlete has gone too high, done too many, or lifted too much.

Gambetta (1992) stated that "training is rehab, and rehab is training." This approach is very true when it comes to the use of progressive plyometric training. Many studies show that ACL injuries and foot and ankle stress issues are the result of too much time spent on the ground and improper landing mechanics. Rather than wait until an injury occurs, coaches and athletes should make proper teaching, training, and performance execution progressions an integral part of the development program. The following chapters provide a great guide to such programming.

Manual Massage Therapies

Yet another popular type of recovery is manual massage therapy, as follows:

- Foam log
- Ball
- Bead
- Water pulsation
- Massage therapist

Whatever the coach or practitioner decides to include in the preparation and process of training for power, understand the ramifications of many traditional yet ineffective practices going on in today's training. Likewise, understand the benefits of proper protocols involving warm-up and efficient training sessions.

Power Training Methods and Equipment

The true art of plyometric training lies in the protocols involved in using well-balanced and well-executed training. These protocols guide participants and coaches through progressions that develop optimal performance and skills.

GEARING UP FOR PLYOMETRICS

Whether you are a participant or a coach, you should keep plyometric training principles in mind as you evaluate your teaching, learning, and testing. Basic progressions and assessment procedures provide good training and lead to the use of more complex training methodologies.

Form and Execution

Proper form and execution are best evaluated by assessing the posture, balance, stability, and mobility of each exercise repetition. Is the exercise performed with upright postural control? Is the movement balanced on the instep of the support foot? Is the movement stabilized throughout all the joints involved? And, is the movement performed with the optimal range of motion (mobility)?

This section provides guidelines for executing the majority of the plyometric jumping, bounding, and hopping exercises. Following all of these guidelines will result in optimal skill performance. Applying these guidelines in an accelerated manner during support-leg coupling, the critical point at which the eccentric part of landing switches to the concentric part of takeoff, is known as transfer of force (Jacoby and Fraley 1995). It becomes the center point of which we can evaluate effective load handling, pretension, and postural control training with, and for, optimal performance.

Toe-Up Guideline

The toe-up guideline involves using locked ankles in slight dorsiflexion, with full midfoot-to-forefoot ground contact upon landing (see figure 3.1). The spring-loading effect of the foot and ankle keeps the foot from pointing or hanging in a toes-downward position. Keeping the toes upward and the ankle locked in a neutral loaded position can reduce the aforementioned effect of slack (see chapter 1) and help pretense the body for better-activated landings. The beauty of being barefoot in early training and learning progressions is that when toes are exposed, proper positioning occurs naturally.

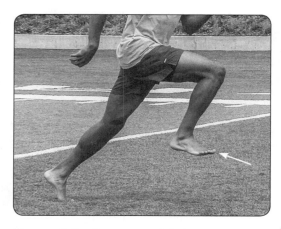

Figure 3.1 Toe-up guideline.

Knee-Up Guideline

The knee-up guideline promotes maximal knee drive and hip extension, or projection. The sweeping or driving of the swing knee forward and thus upward maximizes the distance between this knee and the opposing and extended stance knee (see figure 3.2). When evaluating acceleration mechanics and effective stride length, in almost all directions, we often look for the space between the knees, not between the feet.

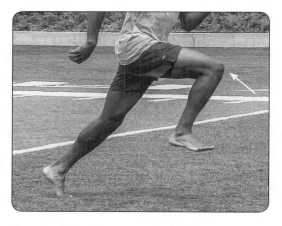

Figure 3.2 Knee-up guideline.

Hip-Up Guideline

When the knees are performing proper upward lift mechanics, the hips can be projected more effectively. Using good postural control and keeping the hips lifted upward and forward reduce slack in the landing system and enhance ground negotiation (see figure 3.3). Considering the body as a stick figure, the more bent segments that exist during ground contact, the more time the person spends on the ground during that contact. When the hips are lifted upward forcing a straighter posture in relation to ground contact, the contact will be more efficient and forceful.

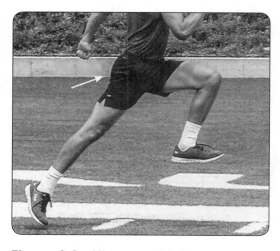

Figure 3.3 Hip-up guideline.

Heel-Up Guideline

The heel-up guideline results in further projection of the hips and body flight by reducing the arc and rate of the swing leg (see figure 3.4). The most common cause of improper running mechanics is that the heel begins to go backward and then upward when the foot leaves the ground instead of upward and forward immediately after takeoff. The heel-up guideline involves initiating lifting and flexing from the hip rather than flexing at the knee. The good news is that when the toes are flexed up and the knee is driven upward and forward, the heel is more likely to move in the proper direction, placing itself directly under the belly of the upper thigh, in preparation for the next ground contact.

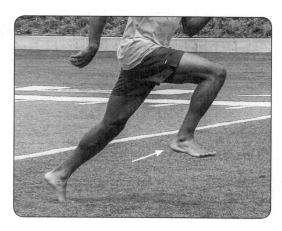

Figure 3.4 Heel-up guideline.

Thumbs-Up Guideline

The thumbs-up, or blocking, guideline is used for upper-body posture and continued force expression. According to Sir Isaac Newton, for every action there is an equal and opposite reaction. When the knees are driven upward in jumping, bounding, and hopping exercises, the equal and opposite reaction is that the shoulders drop forward to meet them. The act of forcefully punching the thumbs upward (as if to poke your eyes out, yet stopping just before reaching the eyes), also known as blocking, keeps the shoulders upright and the torso in proper takeoff and landing posture, and from an elbows-back preparation, synchronizes the summation of force upward, preparing the person for the next takeoff (see figure 3.5). Allowing the thumbs (or hands) to circle up and back over the head slows the entire movement and elicits a loss of force.

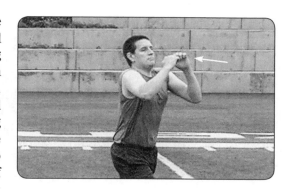

Figure 3.5 Thumbs-up guideline.

Performance Breathing

Athletes need to understand relaxation, especially of the face and neck, to perform with postural control. Using proper breathing mechanics is crucial and can assist in structural support and execution. Following are some guidelines:

• *Inhale during the descent.* Taking a breath in is part of the preparation for takeoff that coincides with the elbows-back-with-thumbs-up guideline and the toes-up guideline for foot and ankle tensing. It is merely part of proper ground preparation.

- *Hold your breath during the stretch phase.* Tensing the joints to create elastic reactivity elements is facilitated by tensing the breathing pattern as well (i.e., holding the breath that you inhaled just prior to landing).
- *Exhale once you have executed shortening.* Breathing out at the execution of a forceful takeoff elicits the completion of the stretch–shortening cycle from both an external and internal standpoint and coordinates, or syncs, the rhythm for continuous movement.

Landing

Jumps with undamped (i.e., without delay) landings produce higher power and force than those with damped landings (i.e., with added flexion and therefore more delay in coupling and contact times). The quicker the person switches from yielding (eccentric stretch) work to overcoming (concentric shortening) work, the more powerful, and safer, the response.

In most cases, a good guideline to follow is to execute undamped landings in jumping exercises. All stretch–shortening cycle exercises should stress active tension upon landing. Clinical studies and practical experience show the value of preparing the musculature for takeoffs upon landing. To minimize ground time and promote undamped, high-tension, optimal-impulse takeoffs, the person should flex the joints and tense the stretch components upon landing rather than after contact with the ground (Bosco 1982).

Foot Placement

Proper foot placement when doing yielding and overcoming work is essential. To obtain as quick a release as possible, an athlete must maintain a locked ankle when landing. Rolling the foot from heel to toe or allowing movement along the ankle joint slows the response and displaces the force from the overcoming portion. The best way to land is with dorsiflexed toes and two-thirds to full-foot ground contact, with the weight balanced on the front half of the foot. One of the best ways to explain this is with the analogy of running or bounding on firm sand. The landing spot should appear to have a large displacement of sand at the front half of the foot and a very faint imprint of the heel (see figure 3.6).

On firm ground and at high speeds, the goal is to reduce slack and improve impulse by loading the ankle in a neutral, locked position and using a short, quick plantarflexion of the ankle (still keeping the toes up). This is the best way to keep the heel slightly off the ground.

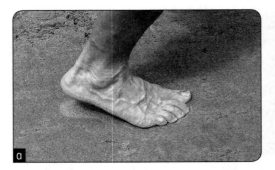 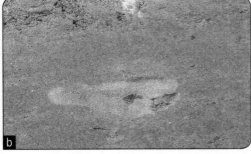

Figure 3.6   Proper foot placement determined by imprints in sand.

Emphasizing landing on the toes or even on the ball of the foot may confuse an athlete and lead to poorly balanced landings and inadequate specificity in most leg and foot movements involving acceleration. As exercises and execution techniques progress, reaccelerating the leg (hip whip) and timing proper plantarflexion of the ankle and foot with the ground to reduce slack optimizes the use of force in the least amount of ground contact time (ankle spring).

Blocking and Upper-Body Synchronization

In all plyometric jumps, hops, leaps, bounds, skips, and ricochets, the athlete should concentrate on the blocking (thumbs-up) rule by adding the arms in a forward and upward punching motion. The block occurs by abruptly halting the motion to maintain upper-body posture and continue force expression. When the knees are brought upward abruptly, as in hopping and tucking movements, the tendency is for the shoulders to drop forward. Holding the hands in a thumbs-up position and executing the block technique counteract this tendency by forcing the torso to remain more upright, thus aiding balance. In addition, the blocking motion of the upper torso can provide 10 to 12 percent of the forces applied.

Follow-Through

Follow-through is important in plyometric movements involving upper-body muscle groups. Continuous force and quickness of action are important. In repetitive throws, such as the medicine ball chest pass or the heavy bag thrust, the recovery or catch phase should not go beyond the point of full extension or flexion. This ensures that limb and trunk musculature is properly stretched (loaded), initiating a more forceful, reactive explosion.

UNDERSTANDING PROGRESSIONS

Exercises performed on two limbs are simpler than those performed on one, especially in terms of balance and stability. Traveling at angles is more complicated from a posture, balance, and stability standpoint than moving in place. That concept leads us to progress from single-response repetitions, in which the athlete performs a single repetition; holds (or sticks) the landing; assesses the posture, balance, stability, and mobility of the move; and then resets and executes another repetition. This style is followed by multiple responses with a pause (i.e., several repetitions are performed with a pause at each stuck landing to assess technical mastery and then repeated without resetting). This helps to condition the body to be prepared for each landing before contact rather than upon or after. It also aids in negotiating the landings better when finally progressing to multiple responses or the true plyometric execution of repetitions in succession and at maximal rate with minimal contact time.

Training should occur progressively along the stress continuum from the simplest exercises (based on the number of landing components, the amount of travel, what happens during flight, and the amount of impact on the body) to the more complex exercises, which tend to be the most shock to the system (see figure 3.7). Beginners should start with moderate exercises, such as in-place jumps and exercises with both legs. As strength and explosive power increase, they can progress to movement exercises of increasing intensity and complexity.

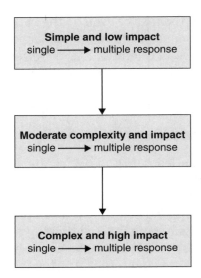

Figure 3.7 Teaching progressions.

Here are a few guidelines for using sensible progressions:

- Focus first on the lower leg and ankle joints (pogo, galloping, prancing, and ankle flip).
- Progress from lower-leg to full-leg, knee, and ankle countermovements (e.g., squat jump, split jump, single-leg stair bound).
- Finally, progress to total torso hip, knee, and ankle countermovements (e.g., knee-tuck jump, bounding, hopping).
- Continue to persuade the body to understand postural control and the differences between joint control in ground contact and that in flight. For instance, the toe-up, knee-up, and heel-up guidelines are accompanied by the thumbs-up guideline for flight purposes, to keep the shoulders and upper torso from shifting forward in an equal and opposite reaction to the knee lift about the hip joint. Upon landing, the toe-up action has a different positioning when understanding the neutral lock and load of the ankle. In addition, the elbows must be behind the torso to further prepare the body for contact.
- With medicine balls, the progression should be from passing to tossing to throwing movements followed by the full multiple-recoil movements of thrusting, swinging, and repetitive throwing.

INDIVIDUALIZING THE TRAINING PROGRAM

For best results, plyometric training programs should be individualized. After evaluating an athlete, training the basics, and observing performance of some exercises, a coach should have a good idea of what the athlete is capable of and how fast to progress. Despite continuing research in the area of optimal training loads, as with so many other areas of sport training, individualizing the stretch–shortening cycle training program is more an art than a science.

Overload and Intensity

A plyometric training program must provide resistive, spatial, and temporal overload:

- Resistive overload—this type of overload refers to the gravitational, inclination, or external stress.
- Spatial overload—this type of overload refers to the range (sagittal, frontal, transverse).
- Temporal overload—this type of overload refers to the operating rate or impulse.

Overload forces the neuromuscular system to work at greater intensities. It is regulated by controlling the height, distance, external loads or forces (or both), and dosage (volume of work) of each variable. Improper overload may negate the effectiveness of the exercise or may even result in injury. Thus, using weights that exceed the resistive overload demands of certain plyometric movements may increase strength but not necessarily explosive power. Resistive overload in most plyometric exercises takes the form of forces of momentum and gravity, using lightweight objects such as medicine balls or dumbbells, or merely body weight.

Many coaches, trainers, and practitioners have tried to fashion plyometric training after some modes of weight room training and anaerobic conditioning, believing that good training is hard (i.e., higher, heavier, eliciting heavy breathing and nausea). Progressive overload in elastic–reactive training refers to the style of contacts and the complexity of the movement, *not* increases in load or duration to the point of increasing coupling time. In its simplest form, athletes can ask themselves whether they are training like a superball or like a tomato. If the answer is superball, the training is smart. If the training is hard, and the contacts are tomato-like, the training needs reevaluating.

Intensity can be describe in two ways, both of which are important to stretch–shortening cycle training. One addresses the amount of force at impact. The other addresses the level of effort while executing the exercises. Following warm-up and progressive lead-up exercises, quickness of execution with maximal effort is essential for optimal training effects. The rate of muscle stretch is more important than the magnitude of the stretch. Greater reflex responses occur when muscles are loaded rapidly. Regardless of the level of progression, maximal effort should be expended when projecting the hips, torso, appendages, or implement. The reduction of impact, complexity, or flight is dictated by the technique and constraints of the exercise progressions themselves, not by diminished effort. Because of the intensity of the exercises, it is important to rest adequately between exercise sequences.

The intensity and amount of overload are two critical variables when individualizing training. Views vary about the optimal intensity and overload for stretch–shortening cycle exercises. For example, many coaches still recommend that athletes need to be able to squat one or two times their body weight to train with certain plyometric exercises. However, as mentioned previously, this does not apply to all exercises under the stress continuum of the stretch–shortening cycle, nor is it appropriate for everyone. As we discuss later, simple tests of progression and evaluation can provide a basis for individualizing the training, even if these tests are not yet based on a substantial body of scientific research evidence.

One notable area in which there is good evidence is the depth jump exercise. Bosco and Komi (1979, 1981) and Verkhoshansky (1967) examined the optimal height for executing depth jumps and found that dropping from a height of 29 inches (74 cm) develops speed. They found, in contrast, that dropping from 43 inches (109 cm) develops dynamic strength. With drops from higher than 43 inches, the time and energy it takes to cushion the landing defeats the purpose of this shock training.

More than three decades ago, Verkhoshansky first addressed the usefulness of depth jumps as an eccentric loading exercise. He searched for a shock method of nerve–muscle reactive ability in a takeoff after jumping from a height. He demonstrated that isotonic weight training marginally improved the speed of running and jumping takeoff. Verkhoshansky (1968) noted that jumps in depth come the closest to bridging the gap between weight or strength training and jump training for speed and that takeoffs after a jump for depth are the leading method of improving the reactive ability of the nerve–muscle apparatus.

Bosco and Komi (1982) reported improvements in jumping ability and increased tolerance to stretch loads in what they termed bounce training (drop jumps). After studying an athlete's behavior under impact (depth jumps), Bobbert and colleagues (Bobbert et al. 1986; Bobbert, Huijing, and van Ingen Schenau 1987a, 1987b), who also analyzed techniques of drop and countermovement jumps (and the force of their impact), recommended choosing drop heights that do not require heel-to-ground contact. They suggested that athletes should land with the weight distributed toward the forward half of their feet, because landing on a flat foot may excessively strain the Achilles tendon.

When eccentric training was introduced in the 1960s, it was assumed that high drop jumps (30 to 45 in., or 76 to 114 cm) were necessary for achieving maximal results (Verkhoshansky 1968). Later, studies recommended that drop heights should not exceed 24 inches (60 cm) (Adams 1984; Bosco and Komi 1979, 1982; Clutch et al. 1983; Hakkinen, Alen, and Komi 1985; Komi and Bosco 1978; Scoles 1978; Viitasalo and Bosco 1982). Our studies (Radcliffe and Osternig 1995) and those of others (Bobbert et al. 1986; Bobbert, Huijing, and van Ingen Schenau 1987a, 1987b) indicated that a further reduction in drop height may be appropriate (8 to 16 in., or 20 to 40 cm).

Volume and Dosage

Usually, the number of sets and repetitions coincides with the type, complexity, and intensity of exercises involving stretch–shortening cycle training. The amount should also reflect the planning stages, the progressions, and the levels of development achieved. Usually, the number of repetitions ranges from 8 to 12, with fewer for more complex takeoff and landing sequences and more for exercises involving lower stress. The number of sets may vary accordingly. Sport scientists in Eastern Europe have suggested 6 to 10 sets for most exercises, whereas earlier, Russian sport scientists recommended from 3 to 6 sets, especially for the more intense jumping exercises. We emphasize that all dosages should be planned according to the continuum of progressive development as dictated by stress and exercise complexity (see figure 3.8).

In the 1970s Russian scientists Verkhoshansky and Tatyan (1973) showed that the sequencing of the high-volume speed-strength training is not statistically significant. This type of training is most effective when matching speed-strength

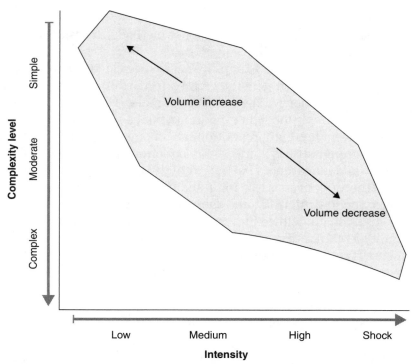

Figure 3.8 Continuum of progressive development.

preparation coordinates with the current functional state of the athlete's body. Sometimes the number of repetitions is dictated not only by the intensity of the exercise but also by the athlete's condition, the execution of each repetition, and the value of the outcome.

Response

Most stretch–shortening cycle exercises fall into one of two categories: single-response exercises or multiple-response exercises. The single-response exercises involve a single, intense effort. Good examples are takeoffs, initial bursts of motion, and releases. Multiple-response exercises, although also intense, place more emphasis on elasticity, speed, and coordination by involving several efforts in succession. One major goal of true plyometric training is performing high-impulse landings and takeoffs in succession. Progressing to the advanced stages of the stretch–shortening cycle and plyometric training continuum requires both types of response. Even better is inserting a third, which we call multiple response with a pause, into the educational setting of the training.

Single-response exercises should be performed with a complete self-check and reset of the posture, balance, stability, and flexibility at each takeoff and landing. Successful performance then leads to executing the exercise in a single-response manner without resetting: take off, land, pause and check, repeat. Because of the no-reset factor, the exercise becomes a continued set of responses, but with pauses. Continued success leads to multiple-response repetitions and progressions.

Again, the main objective of true plyometric training is to perform multiple repetitions in a very elastic and reactive manner. There is little to no benefit to, and sometimes problems with, attempting multiple-response repetitions with slow and sloppy contacts. Therefore, athletes should work the single-response method for the postural, stabilizing benefits and some of the balance and technique requirements, but when using multiple-response methods, they should do them—as often mentioned in this book—like superballs.

These exercises are performed to improve nerve–muscle reactions, explosiveness, quickness, and the ability to generate forces in certain directions. An athlete benefits only from repetitions done well. For example, if he performs a set of hops, bounds, or throws correctly for eight repetitions, but begins to fatigue and performs incorrectly thereafter, then eight repetitions are enough. Given the elastic–reactive nature of this training, little is gained with low-effort, poorly executed exercises. Several coaches and researchers have used high-volume exercises and exercises to investigate the effectiveness of high-endurance elasticity, but the exercises are low impact and low intensity, and they involve low movement complexity. As the basic progression guidelines in this chapter attest, training effects occur as a result of quality, not quantity.

The numbers of sets, repetitions, and rest periods we recommend in the following chapters are based on our experiences of teaching and coaching plyometric training at the junior high, high school, college, professional, and elite levels and on research literature for particular exercises. They are not absolutes, but merely a basis from which to begin and then evaluate and progress. The values within the objectives should be adjusted to achieve training goals. Determining the volume of plyometric training is an inexact science at this time; we need continued research in this area.

Force and Time

Both force and movement velocity are important in plyometric training. In many cases the critical concern is the speed of a particular action. For example, in shot-putting, the primary objective is to exert maximal force throughout the movement. The quicker the athlete executes the action sequence, the greater the force she will generate and the longer the distance she will achieve. As noted in chapter 1, the impulse of the movement is key. Movements must have a high impulse to genuinely train in the manner that the stretch–shortening cycle and plyometrics have suggested. The measure of impulsive action may truly dictate the effectiveness of training and performance.

Rest

A rest period of one or two minutes between sets is usually sufficient for the neuromuscular systems stressed by stretch–shortening cycle exercises to recuperate. Much depends on where the exercises exist along the stress continuum scale. Exercises of low impact and low landing or catching intensity (e.g., medicine ball, heavy bag) may allow minimal rest periods of 30 to 60 seconds, enough time to walk back or change places with a partner or group of practitioners. At the shock end of the stress scale, exercise repetitions may require two or three minutes or more for the systems to be able to handle the forces necessary for optimal execution. An adequate period of rest between training days is also important for proper recovery of muscles, ligaments, and tendons.

The frequency most trainers advocate is two or three days per week of plyometric training, which seems to provide optimal results. It is important to consider the total training load, the type of activity specific to each sport, and the influence of the inverse relationship between frequency and intensity.

Noted authorities (Gambetta et al. 1986) have suggested that the emphasis of the training day be the major guideline when planning workouts. When plyometric activities are performed on the same days as other lifting, sprinting, or throwing activities, athletes or coaches should prioritize their importance. If the goal is developing elastic strength, then the volume of plyometric work should be larger and placed earlier in the workout day—before more relative or dynamic strength work. If elastic strength is of lower priority than other speed or strength work, then the plyometric work may follow those workout activities and their dosages can be adjusted accordingly. In addition, within the training microcycle (week), attention is paid to various strength modalities (e.g., dynamic versus absolute), which can also dictate where to place elastic strength work. Table 3.1 gives examples of workout weeks for programs with time constraints.

Specificity

As mentioned in chapter 1, improving performance requires using the principle of specificity. The dynamic structures of a skill are based on the muscular components of force, contraction, and recruitment. Considering spatial orientation can help with skill development; for example, using positions that mimic the angles and degrees of contraction of a skill improves neuromuscular activity and results in measurable increases in performance.

As mentioned in chapter 1, keeping a good blend of intramuscular and intermuscular coordination within the training is important. Strength and speed

Table 3.1 Weekly Workout Schedule

Sunday	Monday	Tuesday	Wednesday	Thursday	Friday	Saturday
Rest	Warm-up Technique Strength Speed Elastic Cool-down	Warm-up Technique Strength Cool-down	Warm-up Speed endurance Cool-down	Warm-up Technique Strength Speed Elastic Cool-down	Warm-up Technique Strength Cool-down	Active rest
Warm-up Technique Speed endurance Cool-down	Warm-up Technique Elastic Strength Speed Cool-down	Warm-up Technique Strength Cool-down	Active rest	Warm-up Technique Speed Elastic Cool-down	Warm-up Technique Strength Speed endurance Cool-down	Rest
COMPETITIVE PHASE						
Rest	Warm-up Technique Strength Mobility Cool-down	Warm-up Technique Speed Cool-down	Warm-up Technique Strength Speed Cool-down	Warm-up Technique Special recovery Cool-down	Warm-up Technique Elastic Strength Speed Cool-down	Competition day
Rest	Warm-up Technique Strength Speed endurance	Warm-up Technique Speed Elastic	Warm-up Technique Special recovery	Warm-up Technique Special recovery Cool-down	Competition day	Warm-up Technique Strength Cool-down

cannot and should not be separated from coordination and synchronization. Mixtures of intra- and intermuscular coordination are key factors in performance, and the training should have functional specificity to reflect these concepts (Bosch 2005).

These increases become evident when, whether simple or complex, the movements trained are the movements evaluated in testing. Movement aspects to consider when choosing body postures and movement planes are patterns, regions, frequencies, and velocities of the performance movements (Bompa 1993; Siff 1996).

When training for specific strength, speed, and endurance, athletes should keep in mind that stretch–shortening cycle exercises are useful for a variety of phases and to address the principles of overload, intensity, and dosage. Different phases of training require different preparatory, technical, developmental, and transitional methods. Using different progressive levels of stretch–shortening cycle training, athletes can train the general, multilateral, and specific aspects while phasing them in and out of training. Training age, rehabilitation, and the closeness of a competitive performance should influence the timing and dosages of plyometric exercises.

We recommend using the progressive exercise methods to develop the general processes of strength (e.g., the relative and dynamic portions) while moving to more reactive portions with shock methodology (in the advanced stages). The progressions are necessary to foster neuromotor (proprioceptive) development. Then, with complete knowledge of the sport or activity, the athlete can apply stretch–shortening cycle principles to develop highly specific neuromuscular improvements in performance.

SELECTING FACILITIES, EQUIPMENT, AND ATTIRE

Once the concepts of plyometric training are acquired, athletes must optimize their training by deciding where to train, what equipment to use, and how to accessorize. The following sections should help in those decisions.

Facilities

Locations in which to perform exercises involving the stretch–shortening cycle are easily located and inexpensive. Participants can execute great plyometric training in backyards, parks, hallways, and even bedrooms. However, selecting the best situations for proper progressive training programs is essential for safe and effective training.

When looking for a good facility or location for workouts, athletes will discover that Mother Nature was thinking of eccentric-style training. Grass, in our experience, is the best surface as long as it is resilient yet cushioned. We do not recommend soggy, muddy grass or dead, dry, cement-hard grass surfaces. Cushioned hardwood floors, such as those in indoor gyms and aerobic studios, can be used for early progressions of plyometric activities; some rugged surfaces, Tartan tracks, and rubber weight room floors can work. Resilient mats such as those used in gymnastics floor routines also work well. Mats with too much give or cushioning defeat the purpose of reactive landings; therefore, we do not recommend anything softer than wrestling mats.

Equipment

The equipment listed in this section isn't costly. Some facilities provide most of it.

Angle Box

An angle box, made of metal, aluminum, or wood, is a set of angled foot placements for use in lateral movements. The precise angles of the box are not crucial. What is important is that each angle be slightly different from the other three. The bottom of the board must have enough weight, or the ability to be secured, so the box will not move during use. The boards must be of solid construction, durable, and nonslip. You can construct an angle box or purchase one from a conditioning product website.

Angle Board

An angle board is made of wood or plastic, with a metal, aluminum, or solid wood frame. The sizes of several boards differ in height and top length according to the size of the box you use. Standard sizes are a 12-inch (30 cm) base and a height of 6, 8, or 10 inches (15, 20 or 25 cm). The boards must be of solid construction, durable, and nonslip. You can construct a multi-dimensional box using these dimensions, or purchase one from a conditioning product website.

Angled floors have recently been introduced to address the angled landing and takeoff concept. These articulating floors can be set at various angles to provide varied contact negotiations.

Bars

Bars range in size from 5 to 7 feet (1.5 to 2.1 m) long and weigh anywhere from 10 to 50 pounds (4.5 to 23 kg). They usually measure 1 to 2 inches (2.5 to 5 cm) in diameter for Olympic style. Athletes can use lead pipes, steel rods, or lifting bars from weight sets, or construct them from pipes, PVC, or wooden dowels.

Boxes

Boxes come in a variety of sizes, ranging from 12 inches (30 cm) high to 42 inches (107 cm) high. A combination of sizes and shapes can be used, including rectangular and multilevel (drop, jump, and bound). Frames should be of wood or metal; homemade boxes can be covered with a rug, artificial turf, or antislip rubber.

Cones

Cones are either rubber or plastic and are available in four sizes: 6 to 8 inches (15 to 20 cm), 10 to 12 inches (25 to 30 cm), 16 to 18 inches (41 to 46 cm), and 22 to 24 inches (56 to 61 cm). They can be purchased from sporting goods stores, catalogs (outlets), soccer shops, or online.

Dumbbells

Closed dumbbells weighing 10 to 40 pounds (4.5 to 18 kg) are appropriate for plyometric training; those with solid handles are best. Dumbbells can be made of solid one-piece construction, welded, or bolted. They are used as much for dropping as for swinging. However, some advanced methods call for releasing the dumbbell before completion. Dumbbells can be found at any sporting goods or weight equipment outlet.

Heavy Bags

Athletes should have a selection of heavy bags stuffed with combinations of foam rubber, sand, or soft pellets, and covered in canvas or durable vinyl. They can be tube or bell shaped, and they can range from 20 to 120 pounds (9 to 54 kg), like many blocking dummies and boxing heavy bags. They are available at sporting goods outlets that carry boxing equipment or outlet catalogs that carry physical education equipment, football equipment, and so on. Bags can also be constructed by stuffing towels and shot or sand into large laundry or carry-all bags.

Hurdles

Hurdles should be adjustable, lightweight for carrying, and made from aluminum, PVC, plastic, wood, or metal. They should range in height from 12 to 36 inches (30 to 90 cm). Hurdles can be purchased from track and conditioning websites or constructed from scraps from plumbing or building sites or used furniture stores.

Landing Pits

Landing pits that use sand and sawdust in dirt can be found outside at tracks or conditioning areas. Indoor landing pits are placed into or on top of the floor or constructed as boxes of foam padding or raised cushions. Foam pit sizes range from 8 to 15 feet (2.4 to 4.6 m) square. Sandpits can range from normal long jump or triple jump pits to large 5-by-30-yard rectangles. Foam padding is available at sporting goods stores and outdoor and furniture repair outlets. Sand is sold at rock and gravel quarries and by landscaping suppliers.

Medicine Balls

Having assorted sizes of rubber or elastic medicine balls is best, although leather balls are fine with the assistance of a partner. The weight, for our purposes, is 3 or 4 pounds (1 or 2 kg) for single-limb work, and 12 to 15 pounds (5 to 7 kg) for total-body exercises. It is best to purchase balls from manufacturers online or wholesale outfitters. They can also be constructed from old playground or sports balls that are stuffed, filled, sewn, or even wrapped in plastic or melted in rubber.

Steps

Look for stair steps that are close faced (no open spaces between steps) to prevent toes from becoming caught underneath. They should be no more than 8 inches (20 cm) high, 8 to 12 inches (20 to 30 cm) deep, and at least 3 feet (1 m) wide. Suitable steps are found in stadiums and indoor stairwells or can be constructed from wood or cement.

Tubing or Bands

Elastic tubing or bands can assist with accelerated movements or provide safe obstacles for incremental jumping. Assorted sizes and dimensions of surgical cord or solid-core rubber cord are available. We recommend the thicker, more solid styles. Dimensions range from 1/8-inch to 3/4-inch (about 1/3 to 2 cm) thicknesses (ask whether that is the total diameter or the width of the tubing wall). Tubes and bands can be purchased at hospital or pharmaceutical supply outlets or from conditioning product websites.

Attire

No special attire is necessary for explosive power training. Any athletic workout clothing that is comfortable; wears well; and does not bind, hinder, or confine joint movements is acceptable.

Shoes

Shoes for explosive training have received much attention. The comfort, stability, and design of the shoe are considerations, especially with constant training. However, the main issue is proper foot, ankle, and lower leg landing positions. These mechanics should be the most important consideration. Experience and clinical evidence indicate that bare feet and thin-soled footwear may be safe and reliable because they decrease the tendency to pronate, minimize excessive heel contact, and lessen other landing improprieties. The proper blend of exercise surface and footwear that fosters attention to mechanics is what athletes should strive for.

Weighted Apparel

All styles of weighted apparel (e.g., vests, belts, anklets) have undergone clinical and practical evaluations, many with good results. We do not recommend prolonged use of any particular style and advise against using weighted apparel during the beginning and intermediate periods of programming.

Once in the advanced stages of training, athletes should base their use of weighted apparel on what will produce the best results for optimal hip projection. They can use any piece that fits well and provides proper contours and that does not detract from the ultimate goals of hip projection and proprioceptive augmentation. Many sporting goods outlets and conditioning equipment websites sell suitable attire. However, keep in mind that external loading will always increase the coupling time to a point at which contact times will not be elastic and reactive and, therefore, un-superball-like! We recommend that all multiple-response reactive landings and immediate takeoffs be performed without external weight, tubing, cords, and so on. The main reason for multiple responses is to improve the ability to quickly and efficiently negotiate the landing. External loading nullifies this.

Training for elastic–reactive explosive power will always require a progressive approach. Athletes must determine where to begin; how to assess their accomplishments along the continuum of stress, intensity, and technical execution; and where, how, and when to use this training.

Power Assessments

Any program dedicated to enhancing performance needs an ongoing method of evaluating its direction and participants' fitness and accomplishments. To use the stretch–shortening cycle optimally, athletes and their coaches need to know whether athletes' ages, fitness levels, and understanding of safe procedures are suitable for them to participate, whether they are properly equipped (appropriate attire and props), and whether good exercise progressions are in place.

ASSESSING ABILITY

Is serious plyometric training a good option? Before getting too far in planning the specifics of a program, the prudent approach is to look honestly and carefully at factors that could affect safe participation in such intense training.

Prior to starting a progressive 12-week program, participants must have a proper foundation. This includes adequate strength, good fundamental exercise techniques, and an understanding of the risks of injury and how to recuperate from workouts.

Trainers must know participants' ages; genetics factors; and levels of experience, health, fitness, and strength. Those planning their own programs should treat assessment at least as seriously because they are their own trainers! They should look for any limitations that might inhibit progressive development in explosive power training.

Age

Chronological age is an important consideration. Bosco and Komi (1981) demonstrated that the maturity of both the nervous system and the skeletal system affect people's tolerance of plyometric training. Youngsters who have not yet reached puberty, for example, should not participate in plyometrics, especially at intense levels. The continual growth of the skeletal system, cartilage at the epiphyseal plates, joint surfaces, and apophyseal insertions make the extreme forces of some plyometric exercises inappropriate.

The inability of young people to tolerate the high loads of the stretch–shortening cycle can cause confusion because they are exposed to forces during play and sports that may equal or exceed the forces experienced in plyometric training with a proper progressive system. The fact is that kids are vulnerable to excessively hard play, yet not as vulnerable as they are to consistent repetitions of excessive overloads.

We contend that 12- to 14-year-old participants can use plyometric training to prepare for future strength training. This has been corroborated by researchers including Valik (1966) and McFarlane (1982). However, we suggest using moderate jump training with youths. Early progressions of low impact and small dosages, as the guidelines and the continuum in later chapters suggest, are best. Adolescents do not appear to experience any significant response to explosive strength training until after the onset of puberty; therefore, training programs should be prescribed cautiously. Planned progressions are particularly appropriate so that young people receive the many other benefits (e.g., good mechanics, coordination, structural integrity) until maturity and mastery develop.

As age increases, nervous system capability, muscle and joint pliability, and energy production decrease, which makes plyometric training less attractive for older athletes. On the other hand, evidence suggests that decreased explosiveness is only partly due to the natural aging process. Increases in endurance training, a lack of such training, and lifestyle also influence how much explosive power a person maintains at older ages. Continued use of stretch–shortening cycle training in proper progressions and using moderate intensities can be effective for aging athletes, as evidenced by the growing numbers of masters athletes in explosive sporting events (e.g., track and field, weightlifting). As addressed in further chapters, anyone's capabilities can be evaluated and their training adjusted based on maturity.

Physical Capabilities and Health Limitations

Having a good level of overall fitness is helpful in all areas of exercise, and training for explosive power is no different. A doctor's physical exam is helpful. Before undertaking such training, people should have good body weight control and body composition, enough cardiorespiratory fitness to exercise continuously for several minutes or more, the strength to handle their own body weight in movements in all planes, and the mobility to handle movement positions in several ranges of motion.

Several physical areas should be assessed not only when planning training but also to determine limitations. Flexibility is one, especially in the ankle joints and calf muscles, to ensure proper foot mechanics and proper hip set and segmental cushioning. Evaluators should examine posture, noticing especially the use of torso mechanics; pelvic tilt; and the positioning of the cervical, thoracic, and lumbar spine. They should check out balance, torso tilt, and each appendage's joint alignment, as well as the stability of the foot in contact with the ground, stance firmness, joint tension, and coordinated control.

Past injuries may limit a person's ability to perform plyometric exercises. Joint stability and balance should be examined to note any past knee, ankle, or shoulder injuries. As mentioned in chapters 5 through 7, progressive exercises are useful in rehabilitation from injuries. Limitations on explosive training may arise from back or spine problems. Excessive trauma to these or any other areas that cause improper landing capabilities need to be addressed and planning adjusted.

Table 4.1 lists the capabilities and health conditions that indicate a readiness or lack of readiness to participate in plyometric training.

Table 4.1   Athletic Readiness

High athletic readiness	• Foot, ankle, knee, and hip integrity • High range of hip mobility • Stable base of torso • Lean body mass • Knowledge of movement mechanics
Low athletic readiness	• Improper foot and ankle mechanics • Improper torso structuring • Little or no physical education • Sedentary lifestyle • Poor nutrition

Individual Differences

Athletes respond differently to training regimens. Coaches need to be sensitive to these individual differences, and athletes themselves must have some self-awareness. For example, differences between males and females show up both in training and performance. In addition, genetic makeup dictates, to a large extent, a person's ability to improve. Factors such as limb length and muscle fiber type distribution have a direct effect on performance. Both athletes and coaches need to be aware of limitations that can arise in training and development. Although these limitations may affect the rate of an athlete's progress, they should not influence the basic design of the training regimen.

Experience

The training age, or level of experience, a participant brings to working with stretch–shortening cycles can be more important than chronological age. Some athletes who have had several years of experience as competitors, for example, have never trained for competition. Some maturing athletes have been extremely skilled in their athletic endeavors and possess enormous talent, yet bring only an infantile level of training as a base. These athletes can be at high risk if they use poor technique and undertake exercise quantities that their body structures are not ready for. Coaches must determine athletes' technical and developmental levels by using quality training assessments (posture, balance, flexibility, and stability) as described in chapters 1 through 3 regarding core strength, postural control, and pretension.

Strength Training Base

Because a strength base is advantageous in plyometric training, a general strength training program should complement, not retard, the development of explosive power. However, establishing a strength base before plyometric training does not have to be a huge endeavor. An often-prescribed recommendation is the once-used Russian suggestion of being able to perform a maximal squat of one and a half to two times one's body weight before attempting depth jumps and similar shock training. This criterion is still useful as a safety protocol for the extreme end of the stress continuum. However, it is not necessary for the other stretch–shortening cycle exercises used in the beginning and intermediate portions of the continuum.

In our more recent research (Radcliffe and Osternig 1995), we found that some correlation exists between squat performance and depth jump capabilities. However, the significance was so low that any predictions about how well the amount of weight squatted determined jump stress capabilities are negligible.

CREATING AN EFFECTIVE PROGRAM

There is probably no limit to the variety of stretch–shortening cycle exercises. Some imagination and inquisitiveness, peppered with a basic understanding of the neuromuscular processes involved, will allow both athletes and coaches to develop myriad useful exercises. However, it is neither practical nor necessary to identify each movement pattern of every sport skill and design a specific plyometric exercise for it. In fact, only a small number of power movements are key in sport. Chapters 5 through 7 present sets of exercises for these power movements. The exercises are appropriate for all training needs; our explanations and demonstrations add a few insights.

The training sets begin with the simple, fundamental exercises and progress to the more complex and difficult. As athletes improve in strength and performance, they can advance to more difficult exercises. Coaches and athletes should both determine whether the athletes have the skills for properly executing the complex exercises using the apparatuses we mention. Proper planning and evaluation should be used for safe and optimal training progressions to enhance sport performance.

The exercises in chapters 5 through 7 proceed in a progression. Coaches and athletes should use the sequences, cues, and performance protocols as guides while progressing through the levels of exercises.

Training Movements and Methods

A variety of movements and action sequences occur in sports. Some are simple and involve few learned skills, but others are exceedingly complicated. Within the stretch–shortening cycle training, a broad spectrum of simple to complex exercises is available. Deciding which exercises to use depends on the athlete's performance goals.

As coaches and practitioners, we continually attempt to use the proper terminology for types of training. We have introduced several systems for categorizing plyometric exercises based on functional anatomy, their relationship with athletic movements, and competitive events.

In this and chapter 5 we categorize the exercises based on the musculature involved and how it relates to particular sport movements. We examine the major muscle groups used in movements and the biomechanics basic to many sports, and we provide a rationale for using certain exercises, and their respective terminology, to train progressively for more power.

Targeted Muscle Groups

The exercises here and in following three chapters are organized along the stress continuum according to three body regions: upper body (chest, shoulders, shoulder girdle, and arms); trunk (midsection); and lower body (legs and hips). Although we consider them separately here, these categories are functionally integrated; they are parts of what we often refer to as the power chain.

Movements and the Power Chain

Most athletic movement originates from the hips and legs. This is true for running, throwing, and jumping actions, which may be the final performance objective or a component of more complex movements. For example, often the energy of motion for the hips and legs transfers up through the midsection in the actions of flexing, extending, twisting, and bending. The upper body finally receives the energy to execute some type of skilled movement involving the shoulders, chest, and arms. The overlying concept in all athletic development is synchronization. The better the athlete can coordinate the limbs across and through the body's core, the stronger, faster, more agile, and more powerful he will be. Throughout this book we emphasize the overall importance of honing the synchronization of movement skills in each exercise and progression sequence.

We have grouped the basic exercises for the legs and hips into jumps, bounds and skips, and hops. Within each category, we present the exercises in a continuum from low intensity to moderate, high, and shock. Table 4.2 is a summary of the basic exercises for the legs and hips. Each includes a description that outlines its purpose, starting position, and action sequence.

Table 4.2 Plyometric Exercise Continuum Scale

Low	Moderate	High	Shock
UPPER BODY (TOSSES, PASSES, AND THROWS)			
Medicine ball chest pass	Chest push		
Wall push-off	Bench push-off	Drop push-up	
Sit-up throw	Arm swing		
Shovel toss	Scoop toss	Multiple hops to toss	
Supine one-arm throw	Kneeling two-arm throw	Stepping two-arm throw	
Supine two-arm throw	Standing two-arm throw		Catch and throw
	Heavy bag thrust	Multiple hops to throw	
	Heavy bag stroke		
Push press	Push jerk	Split jerk	
CORE (TWISTS, SWINGS, AND WHIPS)			
Medicine ball over under	Leg toss	Vertical swing	
Medicine ball half twist	Bar twist	Horizontal swing	
Medicine ball full twist			Twist toss
Lean—pull—push	Bar kip-up	Floor kip	
LEGS AND HIPS (JUMPS, BOUNDS, SKIPS, HOPS)			
Pogo	Double-leg slide kick	Double scissors jump	Depth jump
Squat jump	Knee-tuck jump	Stride jump	Box jump (multiple response)
Box jump	Split jump	Stride jump crossover	Depth leap
Rocket jump	Scissors jump	Quick leap	Depth jump leap
Star jump			

(continued)

Table 4.2   Plyometric Exercise Continuum Scale   (continued)

Low	Moderate	High	Shock
LEGS AND HIPS (JUMPS, BOUNDS, SKIPS, HOPS) (CONTINUED)			
Prancing	Single-leg stair bound	Lateral bound	
Galloping	Double-leg incline bound		Alternate-leg diagonal bound
Fast skipping	Lateral stair bound	Box skip	
Ankle flip	Lateral stair bound		Box bound
Lateral bound (single response)		Alternate-leg bound	
Double-leg speed hop			
Double-leg hop progression	Angle hop	Single-leg lateral hop	
Double-leg speed hop	Single-leg slide kick		Decline hop
Incremental vertical hop	Single-leg hop progression		
Side hop	Single-leg speed hop		
Side hop—sprint		Single-leg diagonal hop	
Incline ricochet			

EVALUATION OF CONSISTENT EXECUTION

All participants should be tested on posture, balance, stability, and flexibility before performing any training. This assessment provides information for planning training level progressions on the continuum.

The following power assessments are useful for all stretch–shortening cycle training movements (e.g., weights, plyometrics, speed and agility work):

- Overhead squat
- Vertical jump reach
- Depth jump reach
- Single-leg squat with foot back
- Single-leg pogo jump
- Single-leg slide kick
- 10-rep bounce
- Medicine ball chest pass
- Medicine ball forward overhead throw
- Medicine ball backward overhead throw
- Jump decathlon

If progress in any area seems doubtful, the athlete should drop back to a previous exercise level or maintain the current level until she meets the criteria. Then she can move onward. Normative data and ranked improvement progressions can also be used to interpret test scores and individualize training programs. Testing at the beginning of certain training phases and then retesting at the conclusion reveal whether the intensity and dosage of the training were correct, too little, or too much. By conferring with athletes and evaluating the intensity and volume of the workload, coaches and trainers can systematically monitor their progress and develop a basis from which to adjust training. Coaches who keep records and share normative data, as we have done in this book, can collectively develop better prescriptions for training.

▶ OVERHEAD SQUAT

Grip a light bar, rod, or broomstick at elbow width and lock the elbows. Hold the bar directly over the head with the arms slightly behind the ears (see figure *a*). The heels of the feet are directly underneath the hips with the toes out slightly wider. Squat as low as possible keeping the heels in contact with the ground and the bar (elbows) locked out overhead (see figure *b*). This exercise can be used to assess and then develop posture; balance; and ankle, hip, and shoulder mobility.

If the bar does not stay directly over the feet, then the shoulders may lack mobility. If the hips cannot sink below knee level, hip mobility may be lacking. If the heels do not stay in contact with the ground, ankle mobility may be an issue.

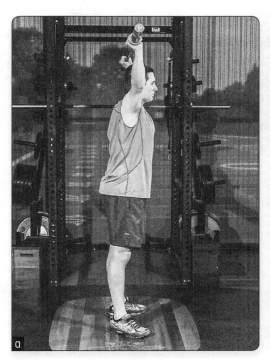
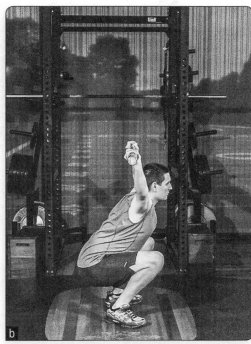

Stand full-footed next to a wall, pole, or measurement device (see figure *a*). Using the tips of the fingers, reach up and mark the highest point possible. Summon all the force possible by executing a short, quick countermovement jump using flexion of the hips, knees, and ankles (see figure *b*); then rapidly extend the entire body and arm reach (see figure *c*). At the apex of the jump, use the tips of the fingers to record the highest mark possible. The distance between the standing-reach mark and the jumping-reach mark is the recorded score.

Take the best of three, four, or five trials. The jumps should be executed without moving the feet before takeoff in a shuffling or stepping action. Coaches often allow a step or even a several-step approach. This test can be used for evaluating specific jump parameters (e.g., approach jumps in volleyball or speed versus power jumping), as long as the validity of the vertical jump test is maintained. The test determines height of rise of the center of gravity. Continually charting these results can offer insight into the form of training that may be lacking (e.g., speed and elastic–reactive versus core or relative strength).

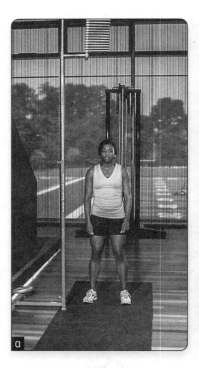 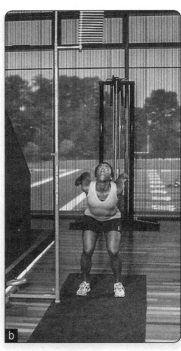 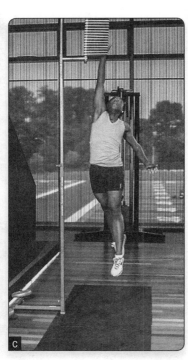

Using boxes of various heights or a stair-step apparatus, drop from levels between 12 and 42 inches (30 and 107 cm) onto grass or a firm but resilient mat (see figures *a* and *b*). Upon landing, immediately jump upward to reach or surpass the mark placed on the wall during the vertical jump test (see figures *c* and *d*). Continue to move to a higher drop until you can no longer attain the same jump height as in the vertical jump. Take one or two minutes of rest between attempts to allow the muscle systems to recover.

This test provides good insight into elastic response ability, and it has also become a popular protocol for detecting high-risk movement and landing patterns. The point of the depth or drop height when maximal vertical jump (rebound) height is attained is the approximate height to train for in this type of plyometric exercise. Practical field work by Costello (1984) suggested that, when performing a depth jump from an 18-inch (46 cm) box, relatively weak athletes jump several inches (7 or 8 cm) lower than their vertical jump marks, as opposed to stronger athletes, who reach or exceed their vertical jump marks after a drop from the same height.

Studies have recommended that drop heights not exceed 24 inches (60 cm). Our studies show that a further reduction in drop height may be appropriate (8 to 24 in., or 20 to 60 cm) as indicated in chapter 3. This and other research suggest that the greatest training effect may occur as a result of prestretch movements achieved from modest rather than large drop heights (Radcliffe and Osternig 1995).

The landing error scoring system (LESS) developed by James Onate and others from research on jumping progression research for ACL prevention (Hewitt et al. 2005, 2006) basically involves incorporating depth jumps into vertical and horizontal movements from a 30-centimeter (approximately 12 in.) box. The LESS score is simply a count of landing technique errors on a range of human movement skills (Padua et al. 2009). The LESS has been documented as a valid and reliable tool for identifying higher-risk landing tasks. Although it may not predict ACL injuries in athletes, it can be useful as a screening tool to identify those who need a longer and simpler progressive training approach.

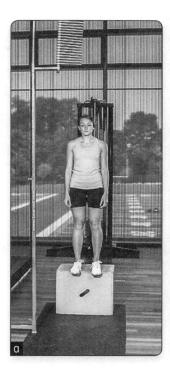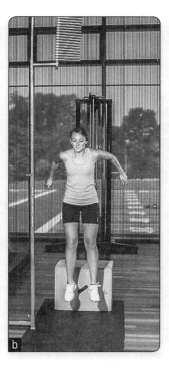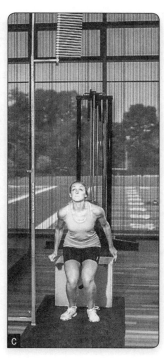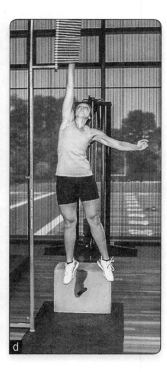

▶ SINGLE-LEG SQUAT WITH FOOT BACK

Lift one foot backward by bending the knee (see figure *a*). Keeping that foot from touching the ground, use the stance leg to lower the hips and squat to a position in which the bent knee gently touches or comes close to the ground (see figure *b*). The stance foot must remain in full contact with the ground. Repeat on the other leg, comparing the two.

This exercise assesses posture by revealing how well the shoulders stay over the stance foot and especially how well the squatting knee stays in line with the toe. It also assesses hip mobility by revealing whether the hip rotates down to allow the knee to touch the ground.

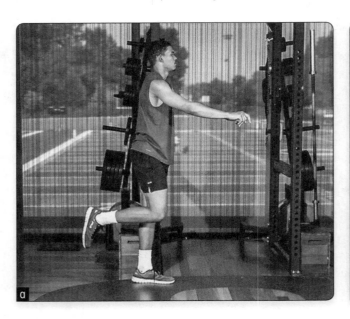
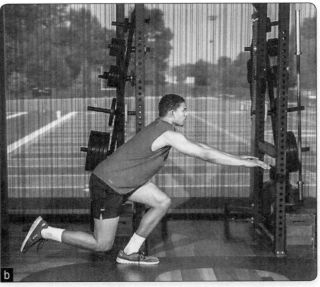

▶ SINGLE-LEG STANCE AND POGO JUMP

Stand tall and lift one leg off the ground until the knee is above hip level, the heel is directly under the midpoint of the thigh, and the toes are lifted up toward the knee (see figure *a*). Perform a vertical jump (see figures *b-d*). Land with the full foot (see figure *e*). Repeat on the other leg, comparing the two.

This test reveals whether you can obtain liftoff from the ground without compromising posture (assessed by the dropping of the swing knee). Also, it shows whether you can land without collapsing the stance and losing balance and stability through the landing joints.

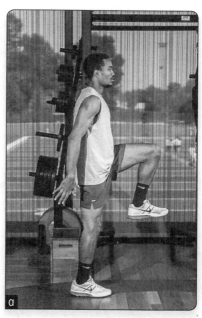

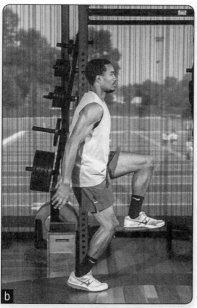

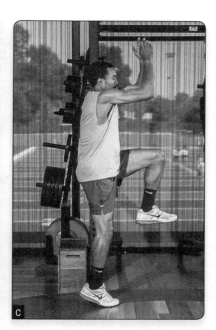

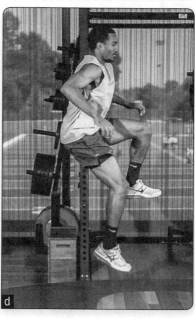

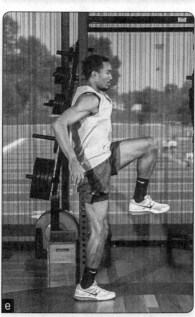

▶ SINGLE-LEG SLIDE KICK

Stand tall and lift one leg off the ground until the knee is above hip level, the heel is directly under the midpoint of the thigh, and the toes are lifted up toward the knee (see figure *a*). Perform a vertical jump and, while in the air, bring the foot up into a position that matches that of the flexed leg (see figures *b-f*). Bring the leg back down to a postural, balanced, stable landing. Repeat on the other leg, comparing the two.

This test assesses whether you can obtain liftoff from the ground without compromising posture (assessed by the dropping of the swing knee). It also assesses whether you can land without collapsing the stance and losing balance and stability through the landing joints, and whether you can repeat the sequence multiple times (three to five) while remaining true to form.

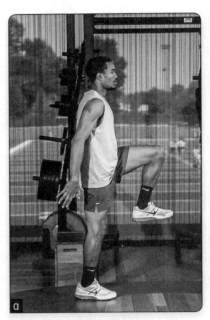

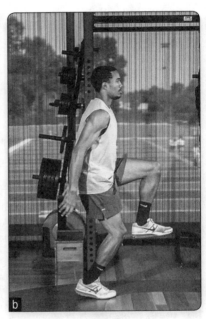

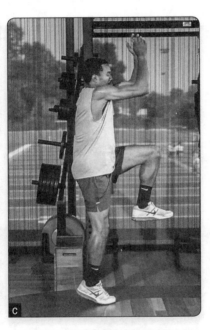

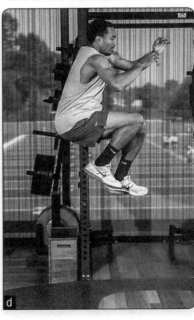

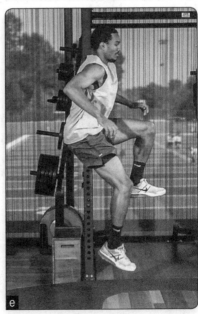

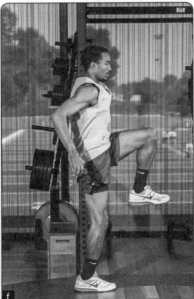

10-REP BOUNCE

Using a contact mat or ground contact testing device, stand with a slight flexion at the knee and the elbows back. Upon takeoff, thrust the thumbs upward and extend the legs to project the hips as high in the air as possible (see figures *a* and *b*). The ankle must lock the foot into a toe-up, neutral ankle position. The spring-loaded ankle is ready for a quick, powerful plantar-flexed takeoff upon landing. Maintain this locked position throughout to ensure sturdy front-half-of-the-foot contacts and quick, elastic takeoffs and a specified number (usually 7 to 10) of bouncing jumps of optimal height and minimal contact time. This assessment reveals the ability to spring-load the ankle, force production and air time, and the amount of contact time.

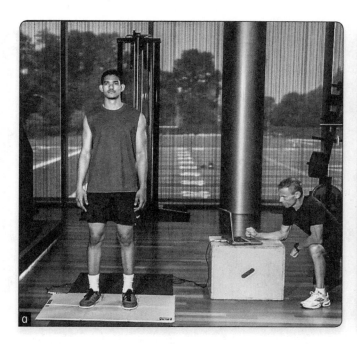

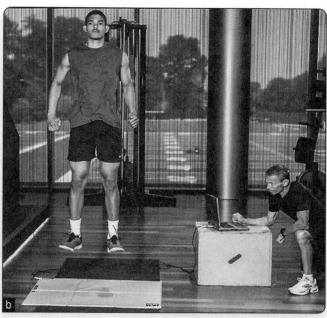

MEDICINE BALL CHEST PASS

Stand with the toes of both feet behind the takeoff line that represents the start of the measurement tape. With a medicine ball of 7, 9, or 11 pounds (3, 4, or 5 kg) placed in front of the hands with thumbs upward and the elbows below and behind, perform a chest pass using as much force as possible (see figures *a* and *b*). The pass is executed by projecting the hips upward and forward and propelling the body forward over and past the start line (see figure *c*).

The distance from the starting line to the ball's landing point can be used as to determine how heavy a ball to use for training. Any passes shorter than 30 feet (9 m) indicate a need for training with a lighter medicine ball. Assess the appropriate weight of the ball by considering explosive capabilities—a ball that is too heavy decreases the ability to impart speed; one that is too light gives a false sense of power output. Use the appropriate size ball for pre- and posttesting to best assess improvement.

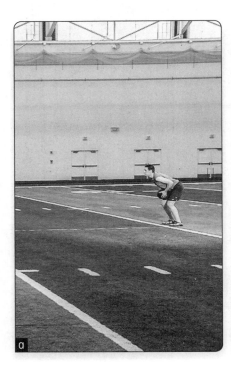
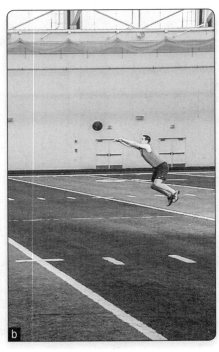
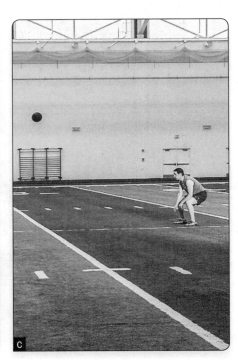

MEDICINE BALL FORWARD OVERHEAD THROW

Assume a square stance with the toes of both feet on a line and hold the ball over the head and slightly behind it (see figure *a*). Flex the knees out over the toes and arch farther backward with the ball (see figure *b*). Then extend the body forward, whipping the hips, shoulders, elbows, and wrists with such force that the feet come off the ground as you propel the ball forward (see figures *c-e*).

Record the distance and rank against previous norms. Assess the appropriate weight of the ball by considering explosive capabilities—a ball that is too heavy decreases the ability to impart speed; one that is too light gives a false sense of power output. Use the appropriate size ball for pre- and posttesting to best assess improvement.

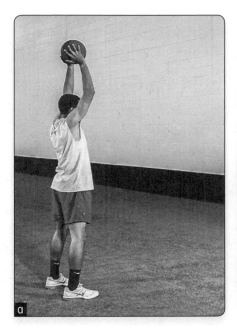

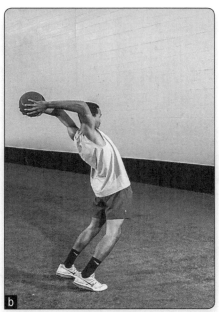

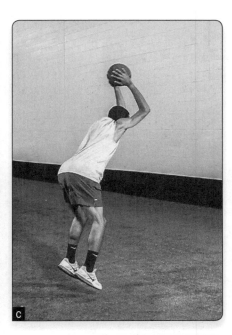

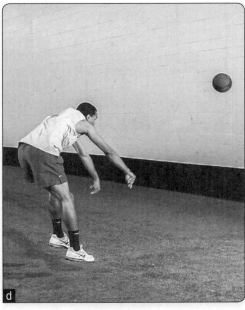

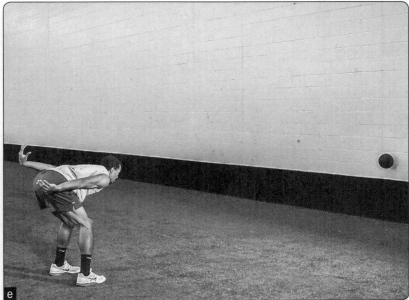

MEDICINE BALL BACKWARD OVERHEAD THROW

Assume a square stance with the heels of both feet on a line and hold the ball below the hips with the arms long. Flex the knees out over the toes and arch the shoulders farther forward, lowering the ball (see figure *a*). Then extend the body backward, whipping the hips, shoulders, elbows, and wrists with such force that the feet come off the ground as both the ball and the body are propelled backward (see figures *b* and *c*).

Record the distance and rank against previous norms. Assess the appropriate weight of the ball by considering explosive capabilities—a ball that is too heavy decreases the ability to impart speed; one that is too light gives a false sense of power output. Use the appropriate size ball for pre- and posttesting to best assess improvement.

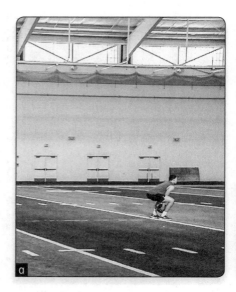
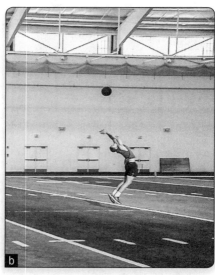
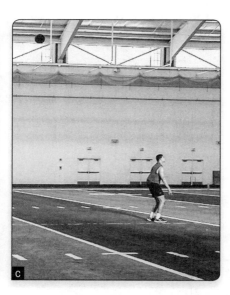

JUMP DECATHLON

A jump decathlon is one way to determine how much or where particular training is needed. This is also a good training session for any athlete seeking to train intensely for power (Paish 1968).

Jump Decathlon Exercises

The 10 jumps in this skillathon were selected because they assess elastic–reactive improvement in a valid and reliable manner. They show areas that lack speed, strength, or agility and coordination so that athletes can work on those weaknesses. These takeoff, flight, and landing exercises are arranged to provide work, fun, and a standardized means for testing progressive capabilities. The exercises are not listed in any particular order.

○ *Standing Long Jump*

Make the standing long jump with both feet together, using the arms to aid in lift. With a quick countermovement of the torso, explode upward and outward to attain maximal hip distance before bringing the feet back under and in front to stick the landing. Measure to the nearest point of contact.

○ *Standing Triple Jump*

The standing triple jump is performed with the takeoff foot in flat contact with the ground and the noncontact leg able to swing freely. This rule also applies to the other hop and step combinations. Take off from one foot to a landing on the same foot (hop); then immediately take off from that foot outward onto the other foot (step). Finally, immediately take off outward and forward to land on both feet (jump).

○ *Two Hops, Step, and Jump*

Take off from one foot to a landing on the same foot (hop); then immediately take off from that foot outward onto the same foot (second hop). From the second hop, take off and land on the other foot (step). Finally, immediately take off outward and forward to land on both feet (jump).

○ *Two Hops, Two Steps, and Jump*

Take off from one foot to a landing on the same foot (hop); then immediately take off from that foot outward onto the same foot (second hop) and then the other foot (step). Finally, immediately take off outward and forward onto the previous foot (second step) and then land on both feet (jump).

○ *Two Hops, Two Steps, and Two Jumps*

Take off from one foot to a landing on the same foot (hop); then immediately take off from that foot outward onto the same foot (second hop) and then the other foot (step). Finally, immediately take off outward and forward onto the previous foot (second step) and then land with both feet (jump) followed immediately by a takeoff outward onto both feet again (second jump).

○ *Five Spring Jumps*

This exercise involves five consecutive double-leg bounds. Keep the feet together and the movement continuous.

○ *Four Standing Hops and Jump*

This exercise starts like the standing triple jump exercise. Take off from one foot and land on the same foot for four consecutive hops; finish on both feet to complete the jump.

○ *Four Running Hops and Jump*

In this exercise the length of the run is unlimited. After a running start, take off from one foot and land on the same foot for four consecutive hops; finish on both feet to complete the jump.

○ *25-Yard Hop on the Dominant Leg*

The 25-yard hop begins from a standing position. In most hopping assessments, the tables are compiled for the dominant leg, although you should test both legs and record a possible mean for right and left. Taking off from one leg, hop for height and distance (leg cycle) continuously for 25 yards.

○ *Five-Stride Long Jump*

The five-stride long jump follows regular jumping rules, except that the run is limited to five strides. Allow two or three successful attempts per event. After a running start of five strides, take off from the dominant leg for height and distance and land on both feet.

Jump Decathlon Results

Table 4.3 (Watts 1968) lists jump decathlon high and low norms results for elite jumpers through those with lower ability. In most cases, the top mark is that of the approximate world record for the event set by professional jumpers of the late 1800s. The mean for the five-stride long jump is from tests once given to specialist jumpers. This table should not be used to compare one leaping exercise with another, but mainly to encourage leaping and bounding as training for other events with a little competitive spirit attached.

Similar to the decathlon or heptathlon performed in track and field meets, such as in the Olympic Games, the distance covered provides a score in relation to the 100th percentile. A score of 100 means the athlete is at the very best level of that event. A score of 5 indicates extremely low in ability in that event. When using the decathlon system during off-season training, athletes should test several of the more applicable events early in the off-season and then retest toward the end of the training period. The main goal is to improve on the *overall* score and one's placement against the 100th percentile.

Table 4.3 Jump Decathlon Norms

	Top scores	Bottom scores
Standing long jump	12' 3"	2' 0"
Standing triple jump	34' 6"	9' 6"
Two hops, step, and jump	42' 8"	12' 4"
Two hops, two steps, and jump	51' 0"	17' 8"
Two hops, two steps, and two jumps	62' 10"	22' 0"
Five spring jumps	56' 0"	20' 0"
Four standing hops and jump	58' 0"	19' 0"
Four running hops and jump	78' 0"	25' 6"
25-yard hop (dominant leg)	2.5 s	8.8 s
Five-stride long jump	23' 11"	7' 0"

Skillathons—A Way to Evaluate

A skillathon is a series of tests and is one method to determine how much or in what area particular training is needed. From research and common practice, the following tests have been selected because they assess elastic–reactive improvement in a valid and reliable manner, and they can show areas in which athletes lack speed, strength, or agility and coordination, thus allowing them to work on those weaknesses.

- Standing and Landing Jump Tests
- Vertical jump
- Depth jump
- Jump decathlon
- Throwing and Passing Tests
- Medicine ball chest pass
- Medicine ball forward overhead throw
- Medicine ball backward overhead throw

At some point, progressions (and progress!) take us from development to refinement. Refining power is not ceasing the development process. Rather, it is an elite approach to the transitional phase of skill mastery, the extreme specificity of power as it applies to the athlete, movement, activity, and sport.

To achieve sport-specific goals, we must determine how much stretch–shortening cycle training is needed and where. We can then analyze performance in the specific training the athlete receives to decide whether to continue at the same dosages, increase volumes, taper dosages, or cease the training for competitive reasons. These assessments and decathlon tables are mainly references to help athletes develop to more elite levels.

Assessing a proper starting point and then progressing from beginning to intermediate and on to advanced and then elite levels of performance are the essence of an optimal power development plan. Knowing what to look for and then how to progress is important for making this training system successful.

Plyometric Exercises

Upper-Body Power Development

Plyometric training is the coordinated use of the entire body in the expression of power. Those powerful movements employ the upper body as they traverse the center of the torso, involving the motions of tossing, passing, and throwing, and their subcategories of swinging, pushing, punching, and stroking.

Tosses and Passes

Tosses and passes are projecting movements of the upper torso and limbs that take place below or in front of the head (or both). In tossing, the functional anatomy is identical to that involved with swinging and twisting, and combinations of these. Tossing by our definition is anything that occurs across the torso vertically or horizontally in which the arm does not go over the head, hence the description of keeping it below (such as forward, backward, or sideways) or in front of (such as upward) the head. Passing is often likened to throwing when comparing the forward pass in American football. However, in our definition, passes are movements in which the implement is pushed from close to the body outward (e.g., the basketball chest pass).

Throws

Throws are projecting movements of the upper torso in which the arms move above, over, or across the head. Throwing employs more cocking and whipping effects than the other projectile movements do, often requiring a start from one side of the head and a follow-through finish over and past the head for maximal horizontal distance.

In many sports, we can see the power the hips and legs transfer through the midsection to the chest, shoulders, back, and arms. So throwing, catching, pushing, pulling, and swinging movements are primarily upper-body activities. Thrusts, throws, strokes, passes, and swings all engage muscle groups of the upper body. The relative degree of arm movement differentiates these action sequences. In their functional anatomy, these movements are similar and involve integrated flexion, extension, and abduction of the arms, as well as the support of the arms and shoulder girdle throughout flexion and extension.

Throwing success depends on how well the transfer of force is synchronized from the opposite foot plant, through the hips, across the body's center of gravity, and up through the throwing arm. Failure to coordinate this load and whip through the hips can cause many problems, the least of which is poor throwing performance. The same can be said about any of the following upper-body-related exercises. A great deal of them are not truly plyometric in execution; however, they are progressive lead-in exercises that foster coordinating and synching the body to achieve optimal upper-body execution of the pass, throw, pitch, toss, punch, and so forth. Using the upper body without this synchronization and without involving the intermuscular aspects sets people up for many forms of failure.

In keeping with the concept of synchronization, we have included the dynamic forms of upper-body lifting, known as the Olympic lift progressions. Pushing and catching a barbell in countermovement style develop strength and speed for overall power improvement. These exercises have been added to the list of progressive work to provide true elastic–reactive training of the upper body.

UPPER-BODY POWER EXERCISES

The following progressive medicine ball exercises are helpful to any athlete exploding from a stance, starting blocks, or a platform (e.g., in the sports of American football, track, and diving). The exercises begin by emphasizing hip and shoulder extension and technique; they then incorporate footwork and reactive work.

1

▶ MEDICINE BALL CHEST PASS

Introduction

Perform this exercise against a wall using a 7- to 15-pound (3 to 7 kg) medicine ball. The movement is specific to the basketball chest pass but is also beneficial in wrestling, American football, and shot put.

Starting Position

Kneel, sit, or stand facing a wall (see figure *a*). Hold the ball chest high with hands slightly behind the ball and arms flexed.

Action Sequence

Push the ball rapidly outward, extending the arms to their full length (see figure *b*). Repeat the sequence upon the rebound.

Variation

Perform this exercise using a partner instead of a wall (see figure *c*).

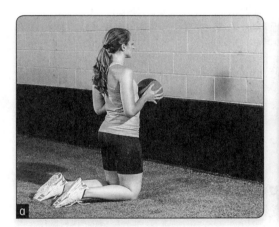

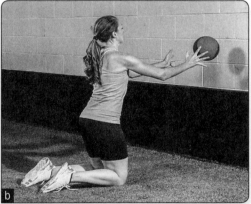

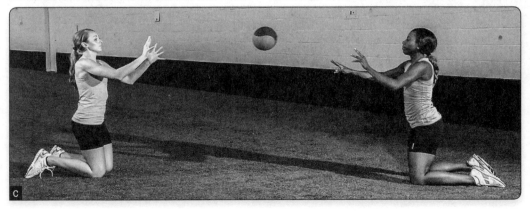

2

CHEST PUSH

Introduction

This exercise is a progressive variation of the medicine ball chest pass. It emphasizes a push involving shoulder and hip extension, rather than an elbows-out, triceps action.

Starting Position

Begin on both knees with chest out and hips high and back. Hold the ball with both hands slightly behind each side of it. Place the ball below the chest with the shoulders in front and the elbows close to the body (see figure *a*).

Action Sequence

Execute the pass by exploding forward and outward with the hips while pushing the ball like a line drive as far as possible (see figure *b*). Correct posture is critical for proper thrust and release. Full extension enhances the execution and provides optimal time for landing on the ground in a push-up position (see figure *c*).

For a multiple-response chest push, execute the pass by exploding forward and outward with the hips while pushing the ball like a line drive as far as possible. A partner or wall then sends the ball back using a skip pass or bounce. After executing the same posture, thrust, extension, and follow-through, immediately resume the passing position. The partner should aggressively skip pass the ball back into your chest. Return the bounce pass as quickly and explosively as possible by catching the ball with both hands and elbows bent, keeping the ball away from the chest and shoulders, and thrusting the hips and trunk forward.

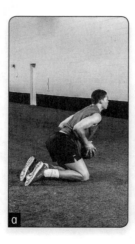
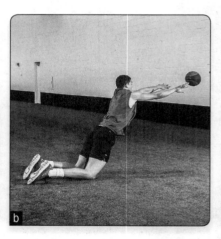
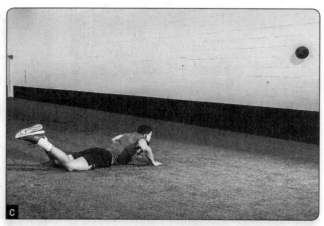

3

Introduction

In this exercise throw a 7- to 15-pound (3 to 7 kg) medicine ball to a partner or against a wall. The exercise directly stresses flexion of the upper torso and applies to all athletic activities.

Starting Position

Sit on the floor facing the partner or a wall with feet interlocked for stabilization. Hold the ball overhead (see figure *a*).

Action Sequence

Throw the ball with a two-hand overhand action (see figure *b*). When you catch it on the return, the momentum forces the torso to rock backward to absorb the shock (see figure *c*). Resist this backward motion with the abdominal muscles and initiate the return throw. Concentrate on propelling the ball with the trunk muscles, not the arms and shoulders. Aim the throw to a point above your partner's head so the arc of the throw is longer, producing greater momentum. Keep the arms extended overhead and do not let the back touch the ground.

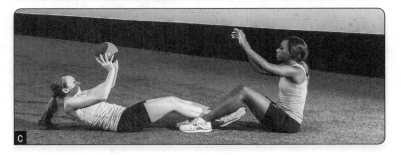

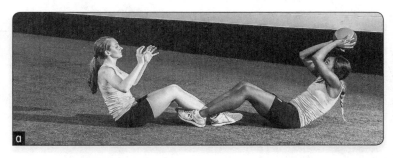

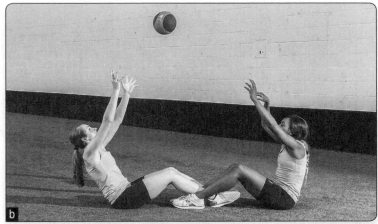

4

SUPINE ONE-ARM OVERHEAD THROW

Introduction

Using a medicine ball to improve overall power production is extremely helpful for many actions, one of those being the overhead throwing motion in baseball, softball, American football, soccer, and javelin.

Starting Position

Lie with the back flat on the ground or a table, with feet flat and knees up. Hold a smaller medicine ball (about 3 to 6 lb, or 1.5 to 3 kg) in the throwing hand (see figure *a*).

Action Sequence

Maintaining a relaxed torso and long throwing arm, pass the ball forward like a line drive to a partner or against a wall (see figures *b* and *c*). Keep the back and head relaxed and on the ground, and initiate arm movement at the shoulder joint without elbow flexion.

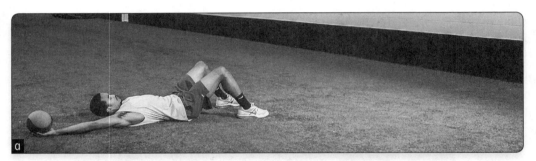

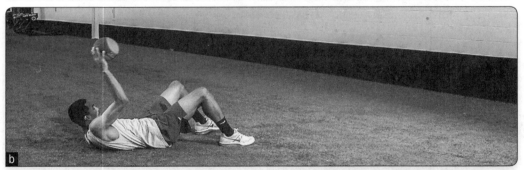

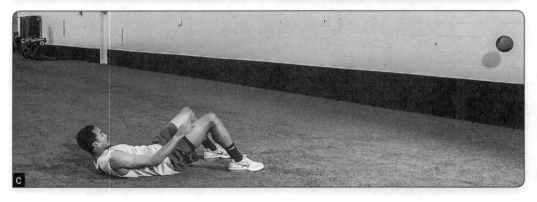

5

SUPINE TWO-ARM OVERHEAD THROW

Introduction

Using a medicine ball to improve overall power production is extremely helpful for many actions, one of those being the overhead throwing motion in baseball, softball, American football, soccer, and javelin.

Starting Position

Begin with the back flat on the ground or a table, with feet flat and knees up. Hold a larger medicine ball (about 6 to 9 lb, or 2.5 to 4 kg) in both hands (see figure *a*).

Action Sequence

Execute the pass by performing a sit-up using the momentum of the throwing motion and the thrust of the chest in the desired direction (see figures *b* and *c*). With arms long and elbows relaxed, the motion is about the shoulder joint. Lead with the chest, and follow through with flexion at the waist.

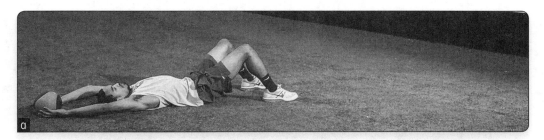

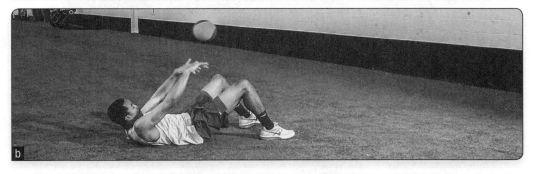

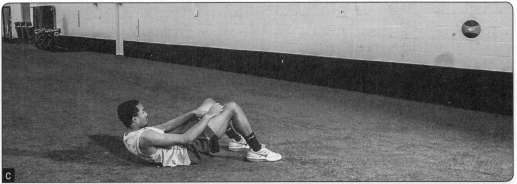

6

KNEELING TWO-ARM OVERHEAD THROW

Introduction

Using a medicine ball to improve overall power production is extremely helpful for many actions, one of those being the overhead throwing motion in baseball, softball, American football, soccer, and javelin.

Starting Position

Kneel with ankles relaxed and toes back. Hold a larger medicine ball (about 6 to 9 lb, or 2.5 to 4 kg) in both hands behind the head (see figure *a*).

Action Sequence

Emphasizing hip lead and follow-through, initiate the pass with a forward thrust of the hips, followed by a whipping action of the upper torso, to complete flexion at the waist upon follow-through (see figures *b* and *c*). Keep the arms relaxed and the elbows slightly flexed. Lead with the chest, and follow through with the shoulders, elbows, and wrists. This is a whiplike action from and about the hips. The hands never touch the ground in any part of this throwing maneuver.

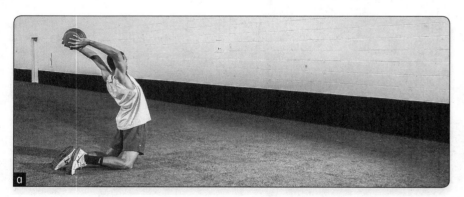

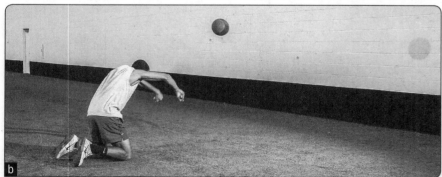

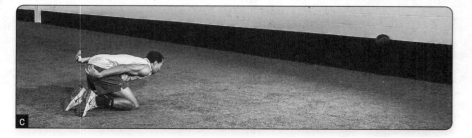

STANDING TWO-ARM OVERHEAD THROW

Introduction

Using a medicine ball to improve overall power production is extremely helpful for many actions, one of those being the overhead throwing motion in baseball, softball, American football, soccer, and javelin.

Starting Position

Stand with feet together and weight evenly distributed. Hold a larger medicine ball (about 6 to 9 lb, or 2.5 to 4 kg) in both hands above the head (see figure *a*).

Action Sequence

Perform the pass as in the kneeling two-arm overhead throw. Initiate the motion with knee flexion, followed by hip thrust, torso whip, and follow-through allowing for a slightly airborne body upon completion (see figures *b-d*). This is a whiplike action from and about the hips. The feet should land close to the same place they left.

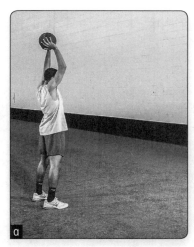
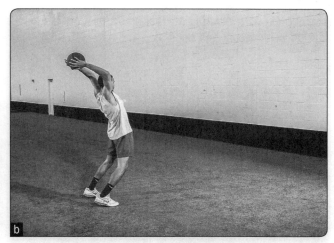
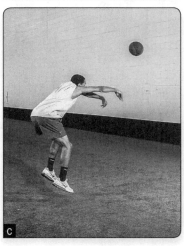
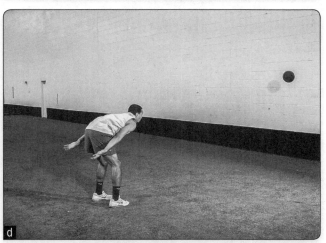

8

STEPPING TWO-ARM OVERHEAD THROW

Introduction

Using a medicine ball to improve overall power production is extremely helpful for many actions, one of those being the overhead throwing motion in baseball, softball, American football, soccer, and javelin.

Starting Position

Stand with feet together and weight evenly distributed. Hold a larger medicine ball (about 6 to 9 lb, or 2.5 to 4 kg) in both hands above the head (see figure *a*).

Action Sequence

This time initiate the overhead throw with a lead step (see figures *b-d*). Step in the throwing direction with the lead foot, thrust with the hip, and whip the torso while pushing off with the trail leg and back foot.

Variation

You can execute this not only facing forward, but also stepping from a sideways position using a rotating hip thrust and open stepping technique (see figures *e* and *f*).

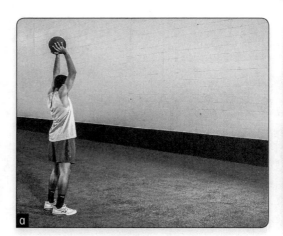

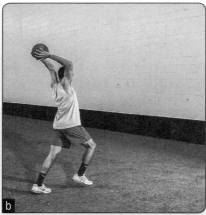

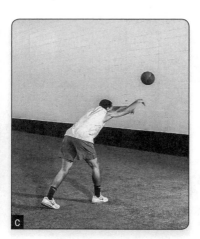

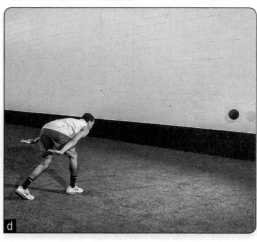

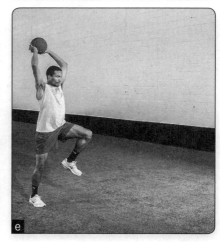

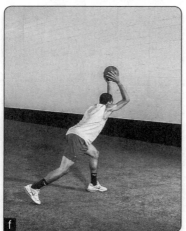

CATCH AND OVERHEAD THROW

Introduction

This exercise represents classic stretch–shortening, or plyometric, work for the upper body because the reflexive response of catching stimulates all the principles of elastic–reactive training in the form of throwing.

Starting Position

Begin with any of the upright starting positions in the overhead throw progression (see figure *a* for an example from the knees).

Action Sequence

Execute an overhead throw as described in the overhead throw progressions immediately upon catching a preceding throw or rebound from a previous throw (see figures *b* and *c*). It is important that you receive the implement in the same biomechanical position you threw from for optimal safety, efficiency, and results.

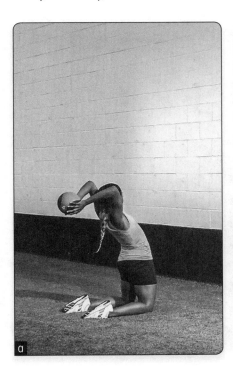
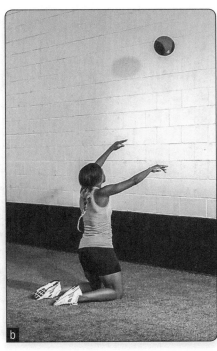
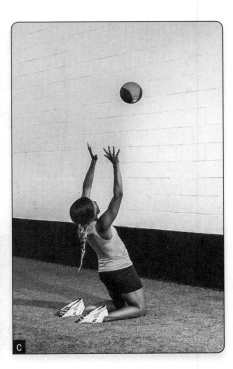

10

ARM SWING

Introduction

Use dumbbells or similar weighted handles of 10 to 40 pounds (5 to 20 kg) in this exercise, which employs shoulder and arm muscles and simulates the alternating arm movement of cross-country skiing.

Starting Position

Hold a dumbbell firmly in each hand. Assume a comfortable stance with feet apart and arms at the sides (see figure *a*). Keep the head straight and tilt the shoulders slightly forward.

Action Sequence

Drive one arm upward to a point just above the head while driving the other arm behind the body (see figure *b*). Before each arm reaches maximal stretch, check the momentum by initiating motion in the opposite direction. Continue this alternating sequence for 20 to 30 swings. Perform a variation of this pattern by holding the dumbbells with the arms half-flexed.

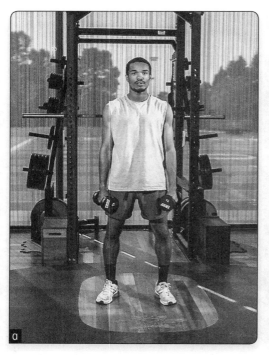
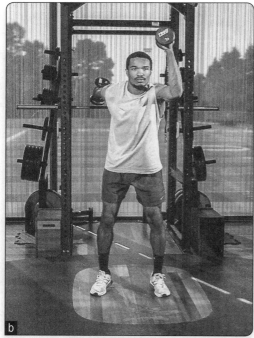

11

Introduction

This exercise requires a heavy punching bag suspended from a rope or cable and involves coordinating the torso and appendages in rotation and extension. It is well suited for discus throwers, shot-putters, American football linemen, and basketball players.

Starting Position

Face the punching bag with legs in a semisplit position; the foot next to the bag is back (although the reverse stance can work for some athletic positions). Place the inside hand chest high on the bag with fingers pointing upward; hold the elbow close to the body and flex the arm (see figure *a*).

Action Sequence

Keeping the feet stationary and mainly using the torso, push the bag away from the body as rapidly as possible, extending the arm and shoulder fully (see figure *b*). Catch the return flight of the bag with an open hand, and break the momentum using the trunk, arm, and shoulder muscles. Push the bag forward again before it reaches the starting position. Concentrate on maintaining the same body stance throughout the exercise. Switch sides and repeat, stressing quickness and explosiveness.

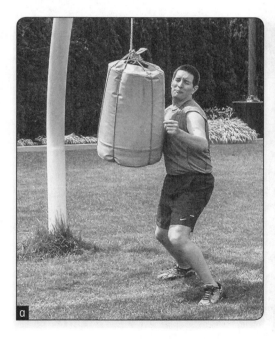
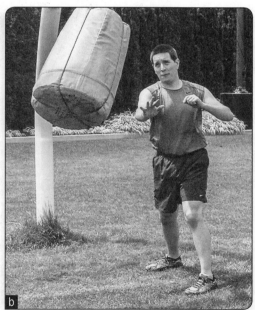

12

HEAVY BAG STROKE

Introduction

This exercise requires a heavy punching bag suspended from a rope or cable. It simulates the motion of a tennis stroke but also applies to training in baseball, discus, and American football.

Starting Position

Assume an upright stance next to the heavy bag. Place feet slightly more than shoulder-width apart. With arm extended, rest the forearm across the bag at chest height.

Action Sequence

Begin by twisting at the waist, keeping the arm extended and pushing the bag with the forearm (see figures *a-c* for forehand and figures *d-f* for backhand). Continue the action until the bag moves away from the body. Catch the bag upon its return flight with the same position of the arm used in initiating the movement. Check the momentum of the bag with the same muscle groups that initially propelled it; then powerfully reapply force in the opposite direction. Remember to follow through, rotating at the waist with each push.

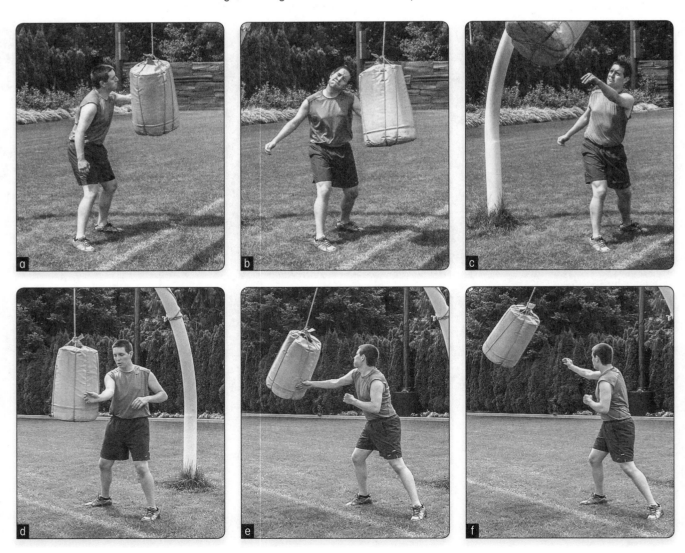

13

Introduction

A lead-in to the higher-impact pushing exercises, this exercise uses minimal push angles and timing.

Starting Position

Stand one giant step from a wall.

Action Sequence

With semiflexed elbows, lean and fall into the wall with thumbs inward and fingers up (see figure *a*). Contact the wall with the arms in position to create maximal extension in the least amount of time. This extension should push the torso back to the original standing position or farther (see figure *b*).

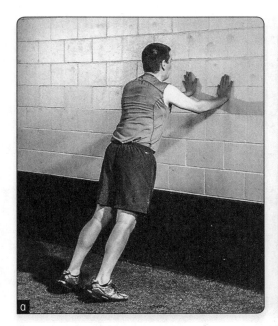
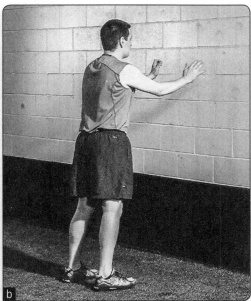

14

BENCH PUSH-OFF

Introduction

A lead-in to the higher-impact pushing exercises, this exercise uses maximal push angles and timing.

Action Sequence

Stand or kneel away from a solid, secure bench or platform (see figure *a*). With semiflexed elbows, lean and fall onto the platform with thumbs inward and fingers up (see figure *b*). Contact the bench with the arms in position to create maximal extension in the least amount of time. This extension should push the torso back to the original standing or kneeling position or farther (see figures *c* and *d*).

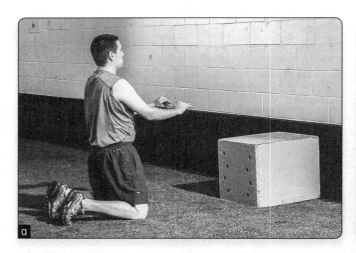

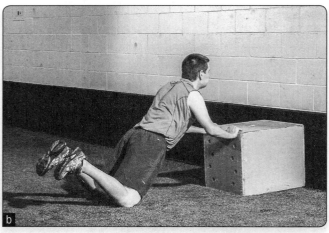

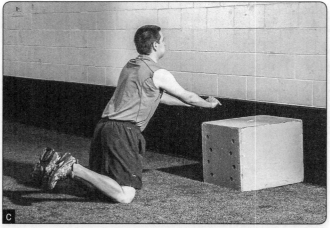

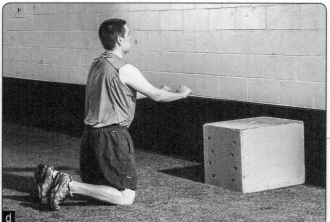

15

▶ DROP PUSH-UP

Introduction

This exercise demonstrates the truest sense of reflexive response and the principles of elastic–reactive training in the form of upper-body pushing.

Starting Position

Assume a prone position with a straight torso, and extend the arms from separate and elevated platforms (e.g., boxes, blocks, benches) (see figure *a*).

Action Sequence

To properly progress, begin by dropping from the raised platforms and landing with a strictly maintained posture, cushioning the landing by giving at the shoulders and elbows (see figure *b*). The next progression is to perform two to four sets of a drop from the platforms and upon landing perform a fully extended push-up. Follow this by a drop and explosive push-up, extending the torso and arms completely off the ground. The final progression is to drop and explosively push the torso and arms back up and onto the platforms for four to eight repetitions.

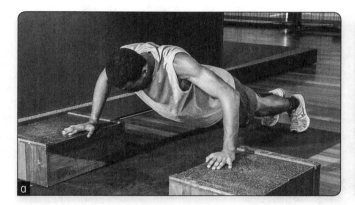
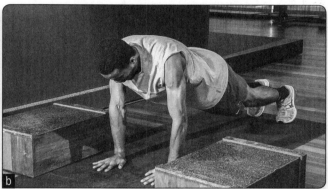

16

PUSH PRESS

Introduction

This exercise strengthens the torso and develops powerful pushing techniques.

Starting Position

Start by positioning the barbell evenly on the back of the shoulders and grip the bar with a pronated grip (palms facing forward and thumbs around the bar opposite the fingers) (see figure *a*). The forearms should be perpendicular to the bar for appropriate grip width. Once familiar with this version, perform the same exercise with the bar on the front of the shoulders, this time with the elbows out in front of the bar slightly.

Action Sequence

Push with the legs and press with the shoulders and arms. Take a short dip by bending the knees slightly to drop the hips (see figure *b*). This drop must be straight down and upward allowing the bar to be projected off the shoulders. As the legs become almost fully extended, vigorously press the bar to an arms-locked-out position (see figure *c*). In the drive phase, the heels may leave the ground but not the toes, establishing the need to press out to finish.

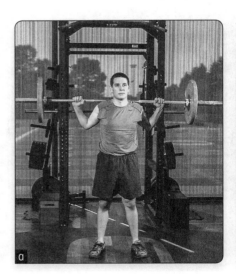
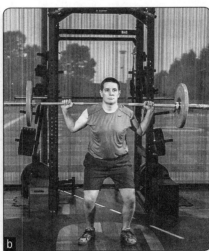
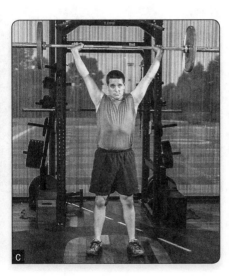

17

Introduction

This exercise strengthens the torso and develops more reactive speed in pushing techniques as used in jumping, shoving, and throwing.

Starting Position

Start by positioning the barbell evenly on the back of the shoulders and grip the bar with a pronated grip (palms facing forward and thumbs around the bar opposite the fingers) (see figure *a*). The forearms should be perpendicular to the bar for appropriate grip width. Once familiar with this version, perform the same exercise with the bar on the front of the shoulders, this time with the elbows out in front of the bar slightly.

Action Sequence

Push with the legs and jerk the bar overhead (see figures *b-e*). The initial execution is the same as in the push press. The exception is that the acceleration used to drive the bar upward causes the feet to leave the ground. The legs and hips accelerate the bar upward. The body is punched into a flexed position under the bar. Move the feet and land in a bent-knee position with feet in full ground contact and arms locked out past the ears. Squat the bar upward to stabilize the weight overhead.

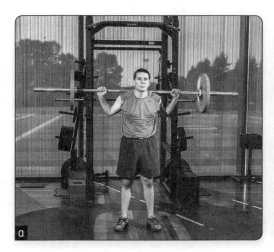

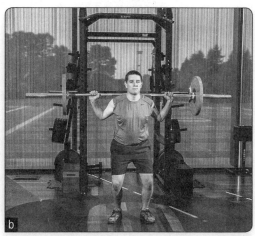

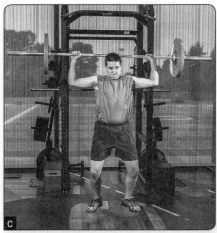

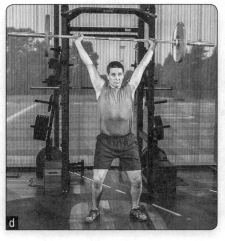

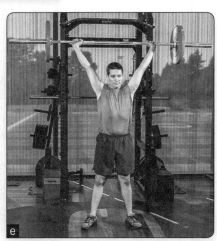

18

SPLIT JERK

Introduction

This exercise strengthens the torso and enhances foot and leg speed pushing as used in jumping, shoving, and throwing.

Starting Position

Start by positioning the barbell evenly on the back of the shoulders and grip the bar with a pronated grip (palms facing forward and thumbs around the bar opposite the fingers). The forearms should be perpendicular to the bar for appropriate grip width. Once familiar with this version, perform the same exercise with the bar on the front of the shoulders, this time with the elbows out in front of the bar slightly (see figure *a*).

Action Sequence

Push and jump with the legs and drive the body underneath the bar by splitting the legs forward and back (see figure *b*). This is the same as a push jerk except that the legs split upon landing and the body drives under that bar and into a lockout (see figures *c* and *d*). The torso remains in the same position as the feet split, with the front foot landing in full contact with the ground. The lift is not completed until the feet are brought back together to full standing.

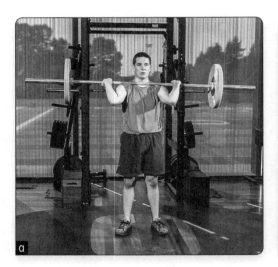
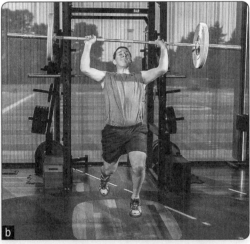
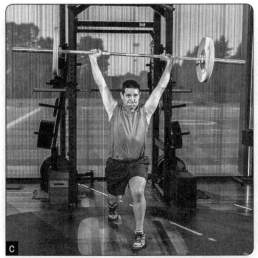
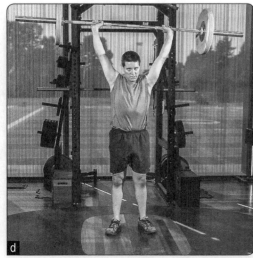

19

MULTIPLE HOPS TO OVERHEAD THROW

Introduction

This exercise combines movements that work the exchange of flexion and extension motions and the subsequent hip projection to help athletes become as responsive and mechanically efficient as possible.

Starting Position

Assume a semisquat stance. Hold 5- to 15-pound (2 to 7 kg) ball below the waist on either side. Extend the arms and hold the head up and back straight.

Action Sequence

Execute a countermovement jump; then extend upward and forward for 1 to 2 yards. Upon descent, prepare the body for an overhead throw backward by positioning the hips over and slightly behind the feet. Flex the knees in readiness for extension upward and backward. Execute the throw with the least amount of ground contact time. You can also execute this throwing motion after a series of forward hops or after one or more backward hops.

SHOVEL TOSS

Introduction

This torso-extension exercise emphasizes the hip and shoulder joints. It is excellent for any athlete who has to explode out of blocks or a stance.

Starting Position

Using a 5- to 15-pound (2 to 7 kg) ball, begin on both knees and place the ball on the ground directly in front (see figure *a*). Keep the chest out and the hips high and back, and position the shoulders in front of the ball.

Action Sequence

With arms long and relaxed, toss the ball like a line drive as far and fast as possible by quickly thrusting the hips and extending the trunk, executing a scooping or shoveling action (see figures *b* and *c*), and then catching yourself in a push-up position (see figure *d*). Emphasize a full extension of the hip and shoulder action, not arm action.

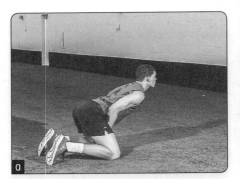
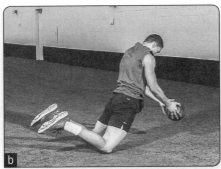
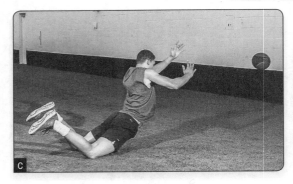
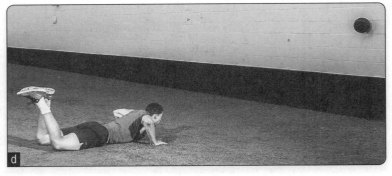

21

▶ SCOOP TOSS

Introduction

This torso extension exercise emphasizes hip and shoulder movement. It mimics the snatch version of Olympic lifting yet allows for a more complete follow-through with the release of the ball.

Starting Position

Assume a semisquat stance. Hold a 5- to 15-pound (2 to 7 kg) ball at or below knee level (see figure *a*). Extend the arms and hold the head up and the back straight.

Action Sequence

Executing a short, quick countermovement, scoop the ball upward, attempting to elevate the body and send the ball for maximal height (see figures *b* and *c*). Distance upward is the primary emphasis. As you land, ready the body to catch the ball on its return down and in front of you. Immediately upon catching the ball, do a countermovement jump and scoop the ball back up and over in the return sequence of the toss.

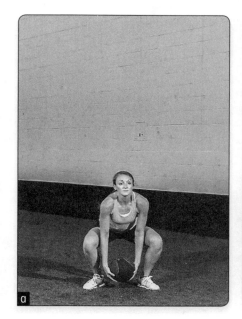
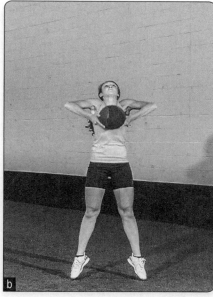
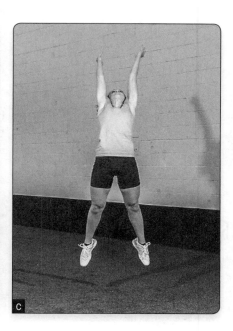

22

▶ MULTIPLE HOPS TO UNDERHAND TOSS

Introduction

As in the multiple hops to overhead throw, this exercise combines movements that work the exchange of flexion and extension motions and the subsequent hip projection. It is excellent for athletes in any sports and events that involve quick, reactive starting movements such as track sprints; high, long, and triple jumps; American football; basketball; and volleyball.

Starting Position

Assume a semisquat stance. Hold the 5- to 15-pound (2 to 7 kg) ball below the waist on either side. Extend your arms and hold your head up and back straight.

Action Sequence

Begin by executing a countermovement jump, and then extend upward and forward for 1 or 2 yards. Upon descent, prepare the body for an underhand shovel toss forward by positioning the hips over and slightly in front of the feet. Flex the knees in readiness for the extension outward. Execute the toss with the least amount of ground contact time. You can also execute this shoveling motion after a series of forward hops or after one or more backward hops.

Core Power Development

In many sports, we can see the result of the power the hips and legs generate and transfer through the midsection. This demonstrates how important the trunk, hips, and legs are for initial power production, support, weight transfer, and balance. Continuing along the power chain from the upper body addressed in chapter 5, we move to the trunk, or torso, shoulder girdle, and shoulders. For our purposes, the structural definition of the trunk is the midsection of the body, specifically the abdominal and lumbar regions. The torso is the trunk of the body including the chest, shoulders, and pelvic region. The exercises for the trunk improve power throughout the torso by developing flexion, extension, and rotation techniques and the posture, balance, stability, and flexibility that apply to all sport activities. Trunk movements include the main categories of swings, twists, and whips.

Swings

Swings are movements of the trunk that are lateral, horizontal, or vertical, with secondary involvement of the shoulders, chest, and arms. Initiated at the hips via proper foot placement and continuing as a rotation through the upper torso, swings are a product of well-timed torque and follow-through. The smooth transition of hip rotation into shoulder and arm follow-through results in optimal execution of the swing.

Twists

Twists are torquing or lateral movements of the torso (or both); they do not involve the shoulders and arms in a major way but rotate the pelvis and spine. Twisting requires being able to keep the feet planted firmly and creating rotational torque with the hips and torso. Once an athlete is proficient in generating torque, the key is to be able to check it, or quickly decelerate it, and reaccelerate it in the opposite direction.

Whips

Whipping movements of the torso are torques that begin by cocking the hips in one direction and then forcefully countering the throw or kip back in the opposite direction by whipping from and about the hips. It is the ability to sway from behind the hips to in front, or vice versa, with a rapid, forceful action.

CORE POWER EXERCISES

The progression of the exercises that develop peak torque and explosive power begin with simple exercises that emphasis foot plant, knee flexion, and rotational hip mobility. They then progress by increasing speed; the complexity of posture, balance, and stability; and the amount of mobility.

Swings

23

MEDICINE BALL OVER AND UNDER

Introduction

The purpose of this exercise is to establish a postural sequence of balance and stability in flexion and extension as a preparation for further tossing and throwing exercises.

Starting Position

Using a 5- to 15-pound (2 to 7 kg) ball, stand with feet approximately shoulder-width apart and your back to a partner or wall (see figure *a*). The feet are flat and the knees maintain a slight bend. Hold the arms long, the chest out, and the hips back.

Action Sequence

Pass the ball back and forth to your partner (or against the wall) over the head and between the legs while maintaining a chest-out posture and full-foot contact stability (see figures *b* and *c*). After performing 10 to 15 repetitions, switch from receiving over (or under) to passing.

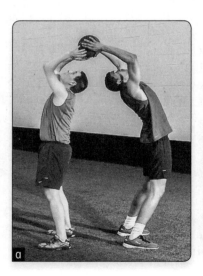

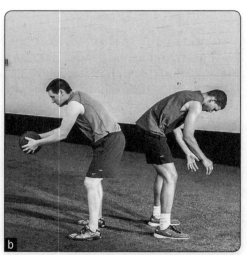

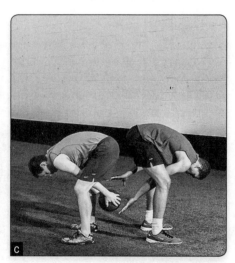

24

▶ HORIZONTAL SWING

Introduction

This exercise requires a 15- to 20-pound (7 to 9 kg) dumbbell, kettlebell, handled medicine ball, or similar weighted object. It is excellent for developing torso power and applies to baseball, golf, hockey, American football, swimming, shot put, discus, and hammer throw.

Starting Position

Place the feet and hips square with the body in a comfortable stance. With arms extended and elbows slightly bent, hold the object at chest level with both hands at arm's length in front of the body (see figure *a*).

Action Sequence

Initiate a torquing motion by flexing the knees and pulling to one side with the shoulder and arm (see figures *b* and *c*). As momentum increases, check the motion by pulling in the opposite direction with the other shoulder and arm. Begin the checking action before the torso has swung fully in one direction; that is, use the momentum in one direction as the load (cocking action) for eliciting a plyometric response in the other direction. Allow the work to come from the shoulders and arms as well as the torso and legs.

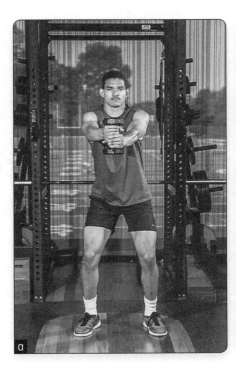
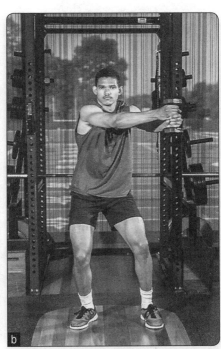
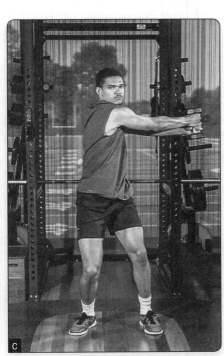

▶ VERTICAL SWING

Introduction

Use a dumbbell, kettlebell, handled medicine ball, or similar object weighing 15 to 30 pounds (7 to 14 kg) as in the horizontal swing. In addition to the athletic applications of the horizontal swing, the vertical swing is beneficial for weightlifting, Nordic skiing, wrestling, volleyball, and swimming.

Starting Position

Grasping the object with both hands, allow it to hang at arm's length between the legs (see figure *a*). Keep the back straight and the head up.

Action Sequence

Keeping the arms extended, swing the dumbbell up and then down (see figure *b*). Resist the momentum of the object in one direction with a forceful braking effort to initiate movement in the opposite direction. In the early progressions of this exercise, the toes stay in contact with the ground for better understanding of the torque involved, eventually advancing to complete takeoffs via extension (see figure *c*).

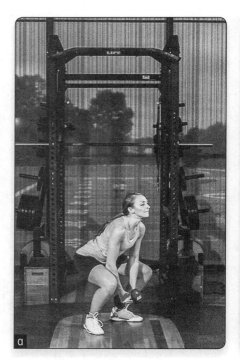
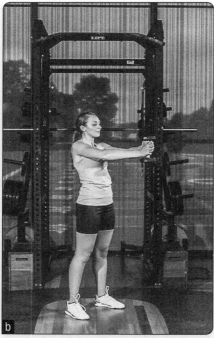
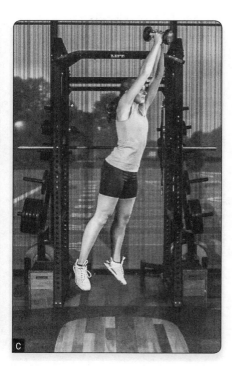

LEG TOSS

Introduction

Equipment for this maneuver includes a 9- to 16-pound (4 to 7 kg) medicine ball and a horizontal crossbar, chin bar, or stall bar. This exercise requires full-body involvement and affects the entire torso and appendages. It applies to diving, American football, gymnastics, and all sports involving kicking.

Starting Position

One partner hangs with both hands from a bar so the feet are just touching the ground. The other partner is several feet (a few meters) away, ready to roll the medicine ball (see figure *a*).

Action Sequence

The partner rolls the ball in your direction (see figure *b*). As the feet contact the ball, catch it (see figure *c*) and check its momentum with a forceful swing of the legs and flexion of the hips in the opposite direction (see figure *d*). This is a whip-from-the-hips action. Concentrate on keeping the legs long and using the hips to generate most of the counterforce. The partner retrieves the ball and repeats the sequence.

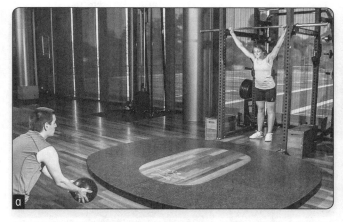

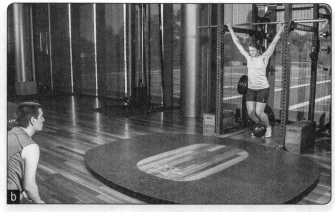

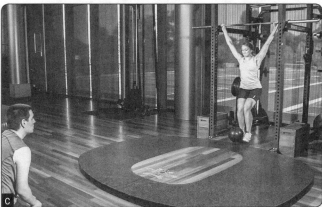

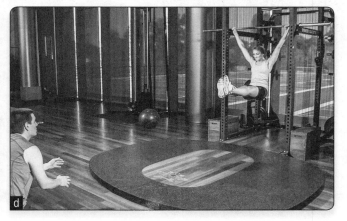

MEDICINE BALL HALF TWIST

Introduction

This is the first exercise in a postural sequence that addresses balance and stability in rotation.

Starting Position

Using a 5- to 15-pound (2 to 7 kg) ball, stand with feet approximately shoulder-width apart and your back to a partner or wall. The feet are in full contact with the ground, and the knees maintain a slight bend. Hold the arms long, the chest out, and the hips back.

Action Sequence

One partner turns and passes the ball to a side while the other turns to the same side to receive it (see figures a-c). Open the hips and turn the shoulders to give and accept the ball. Keep the feet in full contact with the ground while emphasizing posture and flexibility throughout the rotation.

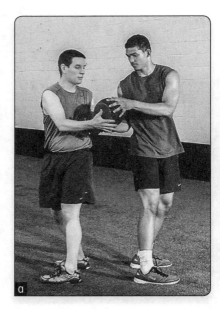
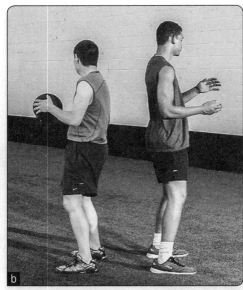
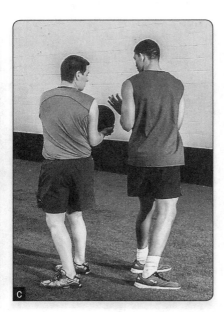

28

MEDICINE BALL FULL TWIST

Introduction

This exercise increases complexity in the postural progression that addresses rotational flexibility.

Starting Position

Using a 5- to 15-pound (2 to 7 kg) ball, stand with feet approximately shoulder-width apart and your back to a partner or wall. The feet are in full contact with the ground, and the knees maintain a slight bend. Hold the arms long, the chest out, and the hips back.

Action Sequence

The posture, stability, and balance tasks in this exercise are similar to those in the medicine ball half twist. The difference is that the increased rotation further challenges flexibility. In this exercise, partners turn in opposite directions, one to pass, the other to receive (see figures *a-c*).

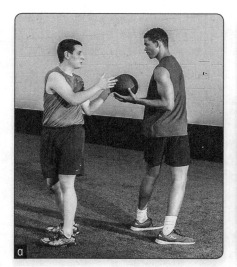 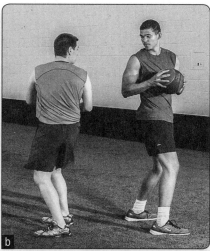 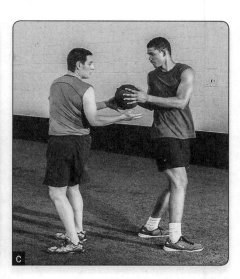

29

▶ BAR TWIST

Introduction

Use a weighted bar of 20 to 50 pounds (9 to 23 kg) in this exercise. Concentrate on using the trunk musculature, with slight involvement of the shoulders and little of the arms. This is an initial rotational exercise involving the ability to counter a loaded movement direction quickly and forcefully. It is extremely applicable to the throwing and swinging actions of American football, baseball, softball, golf, and track and field.

Starting Position

Standing upright, place the bar on the shoulders and hold it securely with both hands as far from the center as possible (see figure *a*). Bend the knees and place the feet slightly more than shoulder-width apart.

Action Sequence

Twist the upper body in one direction (see figure *b*); then before the torso is fully rotated, initiate the action in the opposite direction (see figure *c*). Repeat this sequence, actively thrusting the bar in one direction and then the other. By flexing at the knees and keeping the torso erect, concentrate on using the torso muscles to yield to and overcome the bar's momentum.

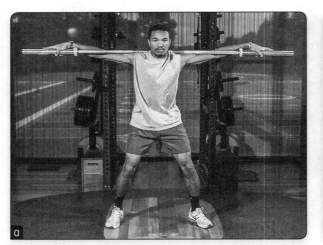 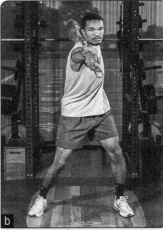 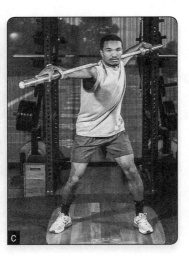

30

Introduction

A 9- to 15-pound (4 to 7 kg) medicine ball is ideal for this exercise, which works all the torso muscles involved with rotating the body. The twist toss applies to training for throwing and swinging.

Starting Position

Cradle the ball next to the body at about waist level. Keep the knees bent and place the feet slightly wider than shoulder width. A partner positions directly to the side approximately 12 feet (4 yd) away and facing the opposite direction.

Action Sequence

Initiate the action by rapidly twisting the torso in the direction opposite the intended toss (see figure a). Abruptly check the initial action with a quick and powerful twist in the opposite direction, releasing the ball after reaching maximal torsion (see figures b and c). Concentrate on using a rapid, reactive cocking action before twisting in the direction of the throw. Use the hips as well as the shoulders and arms.

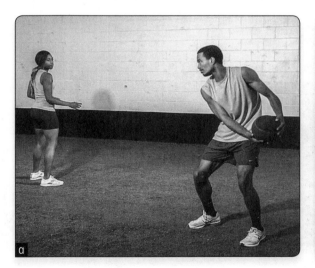

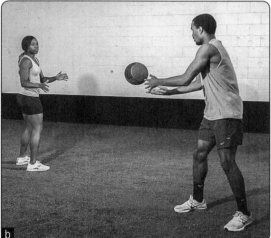

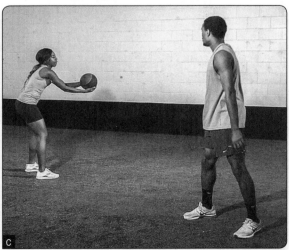

31

▶ BALANCED TOSS

Introduction

This exercise improves balance and stability by employing the skills of catching and tossing.

Starting Position

One partner begins seated with the feet off the ground and balanced on the buttocks. The other faces the seated partner standing upright and balancing on one leg with the off knee held above hip level. The standing partner switches legs after half of the repetitions.

Action Sequence

Begin by standing on one leg with the knee of the swing leg above the hip and the heel just in front of the support knee (see figure *a*). Toss the ball to a partner or at a wall to the front of you so that it returns at different places (see figure *b*). Attempt to maintain this postural position while catching the ball using various twisted positions. Continue for 10 to 20 tosses. The exercise progresses to tossing and catching from positions to the side and behind (see figure *c*).

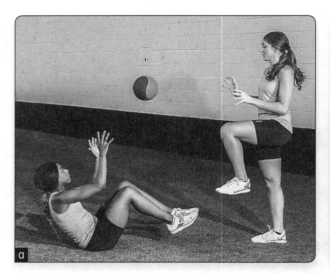

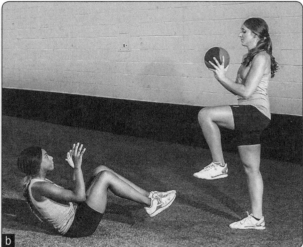

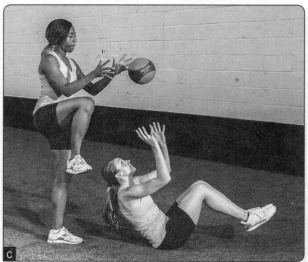

32

▶ LEAN, PULL, AND PUSH

Introduction

This exercise enhances strength and mobility throughout the torso. It is best to use a form of stall bars or an Olympic lifting bar securely placed in a rack at approximately eye level.

Starting Position

Grab a bar that is at approximately shoulder level. Walk away until the arms are hanging at full length and the toes are the only body part touching the ground (see figures *a* and *b*).

Action Sequence

From this full hang, pull yourself up, and, using a snap or whip effect from the hips, push yourself back to a full standing position (see figures *c* and *d*). In the first few attempts, you may feel as though you will break in half. Soon, you should be able to push away with enough power to regain your standing position three to five times.

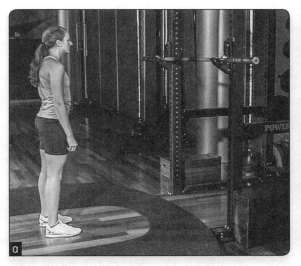
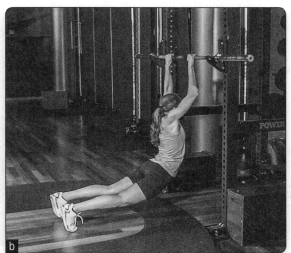
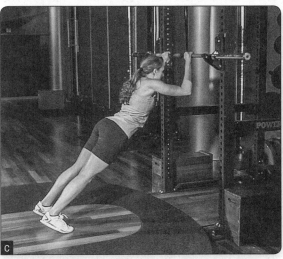
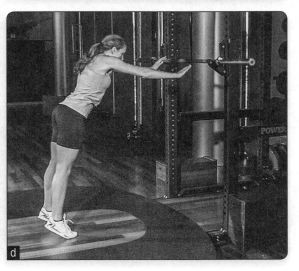

33

Introduction

This exercise enhances strength and mobility throughout the torso. It is best to use a form of stall bars or an Olympic lifting bar securely placed in a rack at approximately eye level.

Starting Position

Grab a bar that is slightly lower than shoulder level. Walk forward until the arms are hanging at full length and the heels are the only part touching the ground (see figure *a*).

Action Sequence

From this hanging position, rock, or kip, the hips forward and upward until the hands nearly leave the bar (see figure *b*). Reapply the grip as the hips come backward and downward to the starting position (see figure *c*). Repeat the kipping sequence three to five times. On the final repetition allow the forcefulness of the kip to launch the body away from the bar and off the ground in forward flight.

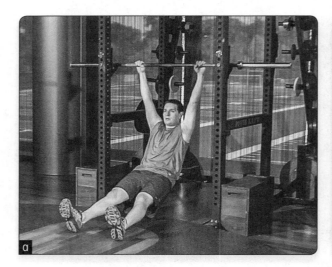
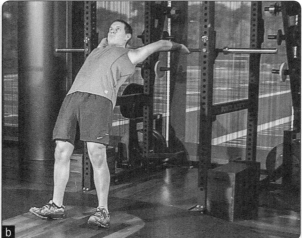
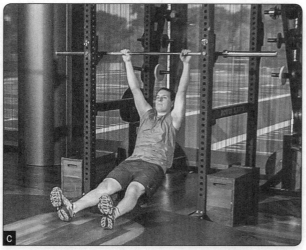

FLOOR KIP

Introduction

This exercise requires a soft, flat surface such as a wrestling mat or grass. The muscles of the entire torso and surrounding appendages participate in the floor kip. This exercise requires a high degree of coordination and explosive power in a total-body effort and is especially applicable to gymnastics, wrestling, weightlifting, and springboard diving.

Starting Position

Assume a supine position with the knees bent and feet on the ground (see figure *a*).

Action Sequence

Keeping the legs extended and together, roll backward far enough to bring the feet past the head as in a reverse somersault (see figure *b*). At the same time, place the hands, palms down and fingers extended, on each side of the head. The body is now in a cocked configuration. To initiate the power phase, rapidly extend the legs upward and forward while pushing against the floor with the hands. Extend the hips and arms forward now, flexing the legs and bringing them under the body in anticipation of the landing (see figure *c*). This is a whip-about-the-hips action. Land in a semisquat stance (see figure *d*). Think of easing into a cocked position from the initial rollback. Concentrate on exploding upward with the entire body, and, once airborne, remember to shift the hips and arms quickly forward.

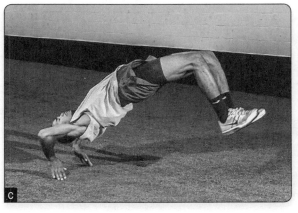
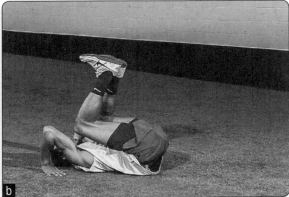
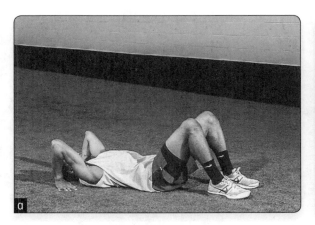
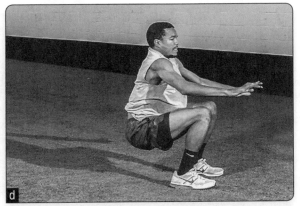

Lower-Body Power Development

Plyometric training was originally developed to achieve more efficient and powerful movement patterns over and off the ground. Athletes were looking to run faster, jump higher and farther, and change direction more effectively, or in other words, negotiate the ground better. Jumps, bounds, hops, and their subvariations (skips, leaps, and ricochets) are all ways to maximize the ability to negotiate the ground and transfer forces effectively in athletic applications.

Jumps

Many definitions of jumping are used in discussions of training and evaluating athletic performance. In jumping, athletes seek maximal height (or in teaching terms, projecting the hips upward), but they may not emphasize horizontal distance. Although lead-up footwork can vary, athletes usually use both legs in takeoff and landing.

Track and field literature refers to jumping as any action that involves taking off and landing on both feet. This is an excellent description, and although it does not fit all situations (e.g., the high jump), it shows another way of connecting training terms with performance terms. When jumping for height, the starting position and initiation methods have significant value.

Following are some distinctive jumps:

- *Squat jump*—A jump performed without a prestretch movement. It is a vertical jump from a static position of ankle, knee, and hip flexion of specified degrees.
- *Countermovement jump*—A jump that includes a prestretch movement. It is a vertical jump following flexion of the ankle, knee, and hip joints and the subsequent extension of the briefly flexed musculoskeletal system.
- *Drop jump*—A vertical jump after landing from a drop of a specified height, the flexion or countering of the landing, and the following extension of that musculature.

Explosive power training includes the following jumps:

- *In-place jump*—A jump in which the takeoff and landing do not involve horizontal travel. Only a vertical displacement of the body takes place. In-place jumps are usually reserved for beginning exercise progressions; in advanced programs they are used in low-intensity and moderate-volume work.
- *Long jump*—A jump used in track and field in which athletes travel horizontally. Takeoffs and landings are of low intensity and high volume, and jumps are recorded in meters rather than contacts (e.g., 30 to 100 meters).
- *Meso-endurance jump*—A low-impact, simple bounding, galloping, and combination jump designed for traveling long distances (40 to 80 meters). Takeoffs and landings are of low intensity and high volume. Meso-endurance jumps also are usually recorded in distances rather than contact repetitions.
- *Meso-power jump*—A jump that involves takeoffs and landings of high intensity and low volume (also from track and field). It involves boxes or alternating or single-leg contacts.
- *Short-end jump*—A jump that involves takeoffs and landings of low volume and highest (or shock) intensity. This jump involves a high degree of complexity and high impact (e.g., hurdle hop, depth jump, and standing triple jump). In the context of explosive training, the shock method was originally meant as a description of eccentric training. More specifically, though, it referred to the explosive–reactive methods involving impulsive types of training (such as depth jumping).

Bounds

The emphasis in bounding is to gain maximal horizontal distance; height is a factor in achieving distance. Athletes perform bounds either with both feet together or in alternate fashion.

In track and field, bounding is any action that involves taking off from one leg and landing on the other. We agree with this definition from the standpoint of the advanced execution; however, early progressions of horizontal hip projection encourage double-leg takeoffs and landings to maintain low stress and emphasize high technical value. Therefore, we place bounding alterations in this category (e.g., prancing, galloping, and skipping) for the purposes of teaching and learning progressively.

Hops

The primary emphasis in hopping is achieving height or distance with a maximal rate of cyclic leg movement. Gaining horizontal distance is of secondary importance early in training, to emphasize the value of the hip projection that accompanies optimal cyclic leg action. Later, de-emphasizing the vertical aspect may become important to accomplish more specific goals (e.g., the hop phase of the competitive triple jump).

In track and field, hopping is described as an action that involves taking off and landing with the same leg. This term is agreeable with respect to the teaching and performance progression. Because of the complexity of hops, early progressions focus on the balance and postural stability required when using both legs for good hip projection and cyclic leg action, regardless of the direction (forward, lateral, or backward).

Leaps

Leaping is a single-effort exercise that emphasizes maximal height and horizontal distance. Athletes perform leaps with either one leg or both legs. Leaping is another description of movements similar to jumping and bounding, usually a single-repetition (nonrepeatable) response.

Skips

Athletes perform skipping by alternating a step-hop on the right and then a step-hop on the left, emphasizing height and horizontal distance. This step-hop method can be applied in all directions (forward, lateral, and backward).

Ricochets

The emphasis in a ricochet is solely on the rapid rate of leg and foot movement. The athlete minimizes vertical and horizontal distance to allow a higher (faster) rate of execution. The plyometric exercises, like many other exercise methodologies, fall under two developmental categories: loading (or resisted) and unloading (or assisted). Ricochets done with the proper feeling of falling can fit into the latter category; some call this the overspeed style of training.

LOWER-BODY POWER EXERCISES

Jumps, bounds, hops, and their subvariations (skips, leaps, and ricochets) are all ways to use the lower body (hips, legs, and feet) to maximize the ability to negotiate the ground powerfully and efficiently. Following are exercises using these actions.

▶ POGO

Introduction

This is a beginning exercise for learning jumps. The posture and the landing and takeoff positions for vertical hip projection begin with this simple lower-leg execution.

Starting Position

Adopt an upright stance with knees slightly bent, chest out, and shoulders back.

Action Sequence

Begin by emphasizing a vertical takeoff, projecting the hips upward for height and using only the lower portion of the legs (see figures *a* and *b*). Use the arms and shoulders in an upward blocking fashion. Emphasize slight flexion and extension of the knee and more flexion of the ankle and foot. Upon takeoff, the ankle must lock the foot into a toes-up position (dorsiflexion); maintain this locked position throughout to ensure sturdy contacts and quick, elastic takeoffs.

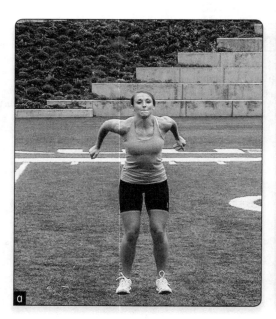
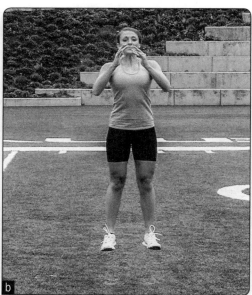

36

SQUAT JUMP

Introduction

This exercise is performed on a flat, semiresilient surface. It is a basic exercise for developing power in the legs and hips and applies to many sports. The primary emphasis is attaining maximal height with every effort.

Starting Position

Assume a relaxed upright stance with the feet about shoulder-width apart. Interlock the fingers and place the palms against the back of the head. This ensures the proper posture for takeoff and landing in the beginning stages of development. Later, when you are regularly displaying good posture, you can use blocking with the arms and shoulders.

Action Sequence

Begin by flexing downward to a half-squat position (see figure *a*); immediately check this downward movement and explode upward as high as possible, extending the hips, knees, and ankles to maximal length as quickly as possible (see figure *b*). Initially, freeze the landing (see figure *c*) and check for quality; then reset and begin another repetition. Progress from the single response to the multiple response with a pause; then finally to multiple responses, initiating the jumping phase just before reaching the semisquat position. Work for maximal height with each jump.

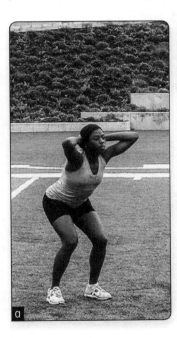 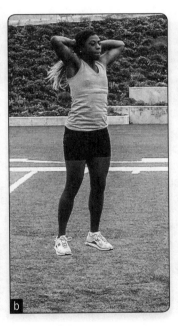 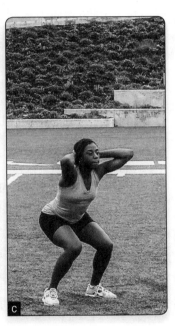

BOX JUMP

Introduction

The purpose of the box in this exercise is to lessen the forces of impact upon landing, aid in executing good landing mechanics, and provide a target for vertical hip projection. Use a sturdy box or platform that is approximately mid-thigh to hip level.

Starting Position

The progression for optimal box jumping relies on an assortment of starting positions approximately an arm's length away from the landing platform, as follows:

- *Static squat*—Adopt a semisquat stance, with feet positioned hip-width apart and arms back in readiness to thrust forward (see figure *a*).
- *Countermovement jump*—Adopt an upright stance with the same foot positioning, a quick flexion into semisquat, and subsequent explosive takeoff.
- *Step*—Leave one foot in the previous position under the hip, and place the other foot behind. Bend the knees and shift the weight to the forward foot to avoid any rocker step action. In pushing off, the back foot creates momentum for the subsequent takeoff upon placement back to its original position.
- *Lateral step bound*—Standing approximately a step and a half directly to the side of the normal takeoff position, push off with the outside foot and lead with the inside leg into a lateral move to a two-foot takeoff from the original takeoff spot.

Action Sequence

For single response, upon takeoff from the progressive starting positions, rapidly extend the hips and knees and quickly and explosively push off the ground while blocking the arms (see figure *b*). Land in a flexed position on the platform (see figure *c*).

For multiple response, upon takeoff from the progressive starting positions, use the arms to aid in the initial burst, jump upward and forward, and land on both feet simultaneously on top of the box or platform. Immediately drop or jump back down to the starting place; then repeat the sequence. You can perform a variation of these responsive movements by alternating the directions of jumping and dropping onto and off the platform. Remember to block with the arms and shoulders and concentrate on minimizing contact times without compromising hip projection.

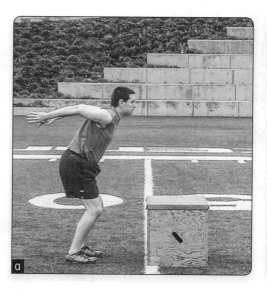 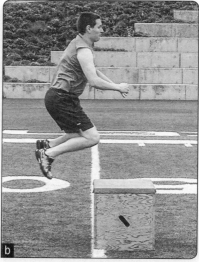 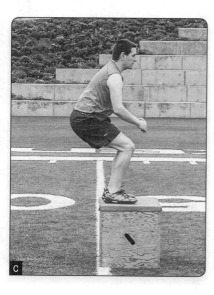

ROCKET JUMP

Introduction

Perform this exercise on a flat, semiresilient surface. It is a basic exercise for developing power throughout the torso and applies to many sports. The primary emphasis is attaining maximal height and vertical reach with every effort.

Starting Position

Assume a relaxed upright stance with feet about shoulder-width apart. Slightly flex the arms and hold them close to the body.

Action Sequence

Begin by flexing downward to a half-squat position (see figure *a*); immediately check this downward movement and explode from this takeoff position upward as high as possible, extending the whole body vertically (see figure *b*). As the body descends, flex the joints so the body is again poised in takeoff position upon landing. Repeat this flexion to full height extension and attempt to stay in one place while repeating this action. Perform this exercise using the progressions detailed in chapter 3: single response, multiple response with pause, and multiple response.

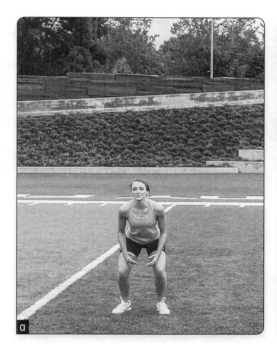 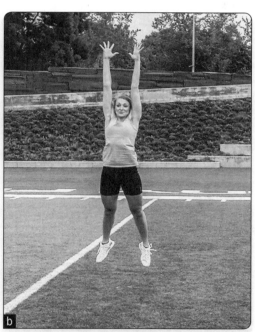

39

STAR JUMP

Introduction

This is a basic exercise for developing power throughout the torso and applies to many sports. The primary emphasis is attaining maximal height and outward extension with every effort. This is a good beginning exercise for work on coordinated movements involving hang time.

Starting Position

Assume a relaxed upright stance with feet about shoulder-width apart. Slightly flex the arms and hold them close to the body.

Action Sequence

As in the rocket jump, begin by flexing downward to a half-squat position (see figure *a*); immediately check this downward movement and explode from this takeoff position upward as high as possible, extending the whole body vertically. This exercise differs from the rocket jump in that the limbs extend outward in four directions (see figure *b*). As the body descends, flex the joints back inward, positioning the body again in takeoff position upon landing. Perform this exercise using the progressions detailed in chapter 3: single response, multiple response with pause, and multiple response.

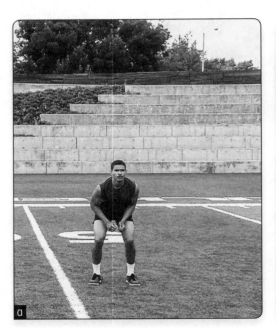 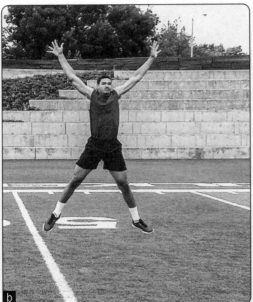

40

▶ DOUBLE-LEG SLIDE KICK

Introduction

Athletes use this exercise as the first of many in which to practice the transfer of force. More forces are applied by following extension with flexion during flight, using the simple act of flexing the knee joint to allow upward lift with the lower leg.

Starting Position

Adopt an upright stance with knees slightly bent, chest out, and shoulders back (see figure *a*).

Action Sequence

Using a quick countermovement jump, extend the hips for vertical height and, upon full extension, tuck the toes up and pull the heels directly upward as if backed up against a wall, thereby needing to slide the heels up to the buttocks (see figure *b*). The knees will rise upward and forward but not in a tuck. Maintain your posture and upright position by blocking with the arms. Perform this exercise using the progressions detailed in chapter 3: single response, multiple response with pause, and multiple response.

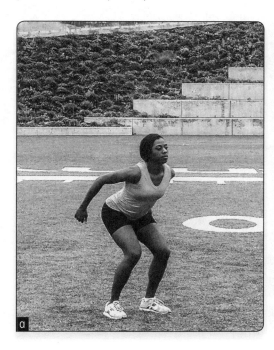
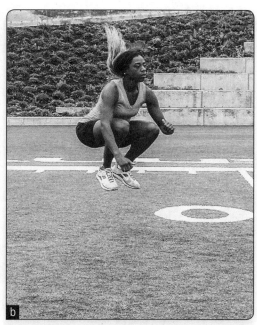

KNEE-TUCK JUMP

Introduction

This exercise should be performed on a resilient, flat surface such as grass or a gym floor.

Starting Position

Assume a comfortable upright stance, placing the hands palms down at chest height. Do this in the early stages to ensure a good takeoff and landing posture and to give the knees a target. Once good posture occurs regularly, observe the thumbs-up guideline as discussed in chapter 3.

Action Sequence

Begin by rapidly dipping down to about the quarter-squat level (see figure *a*) and immediately explode upward. Drive the knees high toward the chest and attempt to touch them to the palms (see figure *b*). Upon landing, repeat the sequence, each time driving the knees upward and tucking the feet under the body. Perform this exercise using the progressions detailed in chapter 3: single response, multiple response with pause, and multiple response.

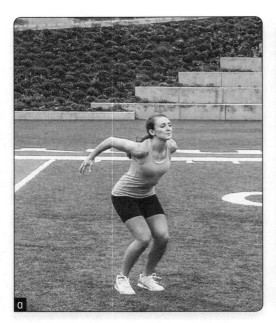

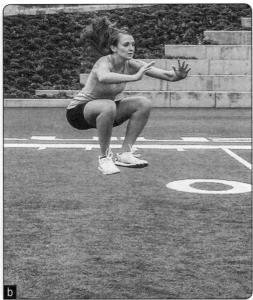

42

▶ SPLIT JUMP

Introduction

Perform split jumps on a flat surface. They are especially good for developing striding power for running and cross-country skiing; they are also specific to the split portion of the jerk.

Starting Position

Assume a stance with one leg extended forward with the knee over the midpoint of the foot and the other leg back with the knee bent and underneath the plumb line of the hips and shoulders (see figure *a*).

Action Sequence

Jump as high and straight up as possible (see figure *b*). Block with the arms to gain additional lift. Upon landing, retain the spread-legged position, bending the knees to absorb the shock (see figure *c*). It is important to keep the shoulders back and in line with the hips to maintain proper stability. Continue the motion for the required number of repetitions; then switch legs and perform the same number of repetitions with the opposite leg forward. Perform this exercise using the progressions detailed in chapter 3: single response, multiple response with pause, and multiple response.

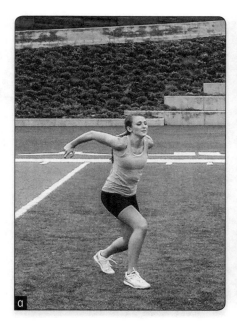 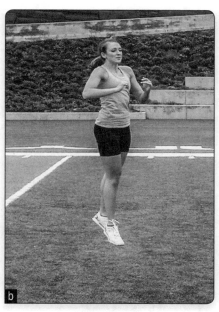 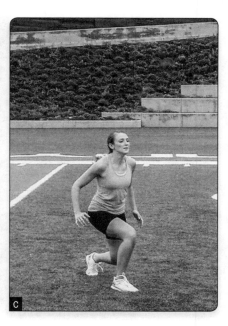

43

Introduction

As in the split jump, this exercise works the muscles of the lower body and torso. It is similar to the split jump except that leg speed is also emphasized; therefore, it is especially good for runners and jumpers.

Starting Position

Assume a stance with one leg extended forward with the knee over the midpoint of the foot and the other leg back with the knee bent and underneath the plumb line of the hips and shoulders (see figure *a*).

Action Sequence

As in the split jump, jump as high and straight up as possible. Block with the arms to gain additional lift. At the apex of the jump, reverse the position of the legs—that is, front to back and back to front (see figure *b*). Switching the legs occurs in midair, and you must do it quickly before landing. Upon landing, repeat the jump, again reversing the position of the legs (see figure *c*). Emphasize attaining maximal vertical height and leg speed. Perform this exercise using the progressions detailed in chapter 3: single response, multiple response with pause, and multiple response.

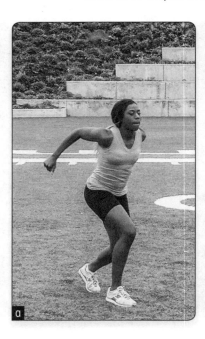
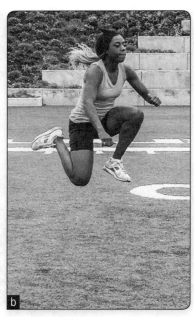
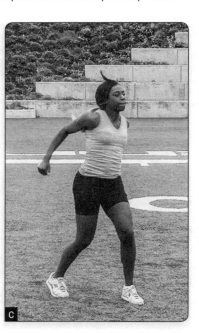

DOUBLE SCISSORS JUMP

Introduction

This exercise is a variation of the scissors jump for more advanced athletes. It is excellent for working the flexion and extension muscles in the hips, legs, and torso.

Starting Position

Assume a stance with one leg extended forward with the knee over the midpoint of the foot and the other leg back with the knee bent and underneath the plumb line of the hips and shoulders (see figure a).

Action Sequence

As in the scissors jump, jump as high and straight up as possible. Block with the arms to gain additional lift. At the apex of the jump, attempt a complete cycle of the legs, front to back, back to front, and vice versa, while in the air, landing with the legs in their original position (see figures b and c). Remember to maintain an excellent shoulders-above-hips posture. Perform this double-switch movement about the hips, involving total-leg movements and not merely switching lower legs or feet. Therefore, perform this exercise in the single-response mode only.

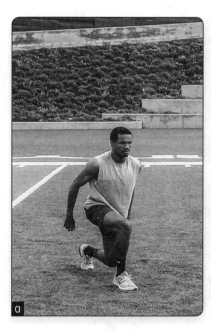
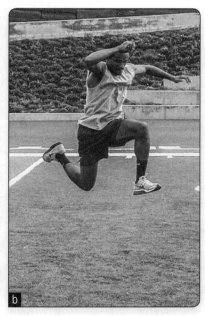
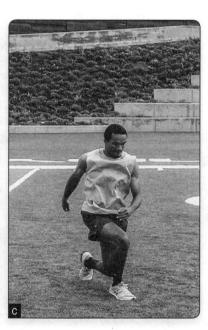

45

Introduction

A long, sturdy bench, rectangular box, or row of bleachers or stadium steps is required for the stride jump. This exercise is excellent for any sport or activity that requires good projection of the hips from a single-leg or alternating-leg movement. The idea behind this exercise is to place the hips and one leg to increase the stride without compromising posture and technique.

Starting Position

Assume a position to the side and at one end of the bench. Place the inside foot on top of the bench, and hold the arms down at the sides (see figure a).

Action Sequence

Begin by executing a push from both legs, simultaneously with an upward movement of the arms. Using the inside leg (foot on bench) for power, jump upward as high as possible and perform a maximal knee drive with the outside (swing) leg (see figures b-d). Begin the training with single responses, focusing on coordinating the downward push onto the bench with the upward drive of the swing knee and arm(s). Synchronizing the swing-and-scissors motion and the step-with-drive motion is very challenging. Perform this exercise using the progressions detailed in chapter 3: single response, multiple response with pause, and multiple response.

For multiple response, repeat the action as soon as the outside leg (away from the bench) touches the ground. Use mainly the inside leg for power and support, allowing the outside leg to contact the ground with minimal time and maximal impulse. Once you reach the end of the bench, turn around, and, reversing the leg positions, repeat the sequence in the other direction. Remember to gain full height and body extension with each jump.

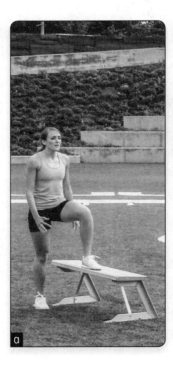
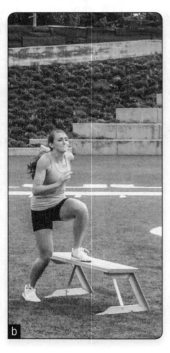
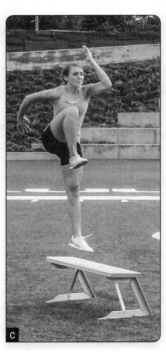
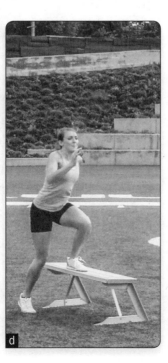

46

▶ STRIDE JUMP CROSSOVER

Introduction

Like the stride jump, this exercise requires a long, sturdy bench, rectangular box, or row of bleachers or stadium steps. This exercise extends the multiple-response effects of the stride jump to enhance running, jumping, gymnastics, and similar sport events.

Starting Position

As in the stride jump, assume a standing position at one end of the bench with one foot on the ground and the other on the bench. One arm is flexed and the other is down by the side of the body (see figure *a*).

Action Sequence

Initiate the movement by rapidly blocking the arms upward. Continue this upward momentum by driving off the bench with the elevated leg (see figure *b*), jumping as high as possible, and extending the body fully (see figure *c*). At this point, carry the body over the bench and slightly forward so the driving leg touches the ground on the opposite side of the bench and the trailing leg rests on top of the bench (see figure *d*). Body orientation and feet positions are now opposite those of the starting position. As soon as the original driving leg contacts the ground, repeat the motion but with the original trailing leg acting as the major power source. Repeat these movements back and forth the length of the bench. Work to achieve maximal height with each jump, using the arms to assist in lifting the body. Minimize ground- and bench-contact time with the feet; perform the movements as quickly as possible. Perform this exercise using the progressions detailed in chapter 3: single response, multiple response with pause, and multiple response.

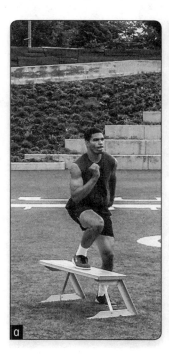
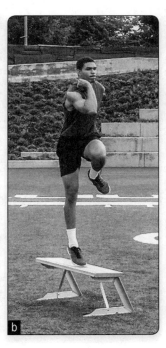
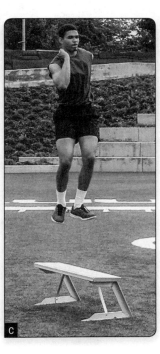
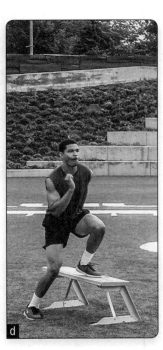

47

Introduction

You will need a soft landing surface, such as grass, sand, or a wrestling mat, and a box, bench, or stool approximately 12 to 24 inches (30 to 60 cm) high for this exercise. It is useful for those in training for volleyball, American football, basketball, platform diving, and weightlifting.

Starting Position

With the feet together, assume a semierect position facing the box (about an arm's length away). Keep the arms at the sides and slightly bent at the elbows.

Action Sequence

Leap toward the box by exploding powerfully out of the starting position with the help of an energetic arm swing (see figure *a*). While moving through the air, prepare for takeoff by assuming a semisquat position, keeping the knees high and forward of the hips, and tucking the feet under the hips (see figure *b*). Upon landing on the box, full footed and with locked ankles (see figure *c*), immediately thrust forward again, this time extending and straightening the entire body (see figures *d* and *e*). Finish by landing full footed on the ground, bending the legs to act as a cushion (see figure *f*). Make the initial jump to the box as quickly as possible with just enough height to reach it. Anticipate and concentrate on the second explosion from the box; stress a full extension of the body after takeoff. You can perform a variation of this exercise by landing on the box on one foot, thus executing the leap with one driving leg. Perform this exercise using the progressions detailed in chapter 3: single response, multiple response with pause, and multiple response.

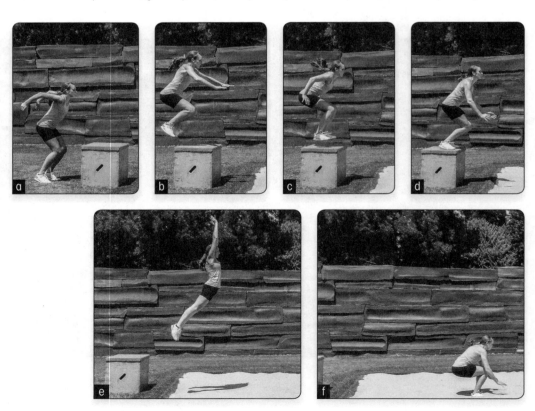

48

Introduction

This exercise requires an elevated surface (box or bench) approximately 12 to 36 inches (30 to 90 cm) high. The landing surface should be forgiving yet resilient; grass, gymnastics flooring, and cushioned turf work well. The depth jump is a shock-method exercise and comes in the final portion of the training continuum. Therefore, progression into this exercise is a must, as well as progression within it. Apply the shock method, which involves a drop or fall from the elevated platform to the takeoff surface. The key is to avoid developing a landing rhythm to work on handling the surprise of landing and the subsequent takeoff. The depth jump is elite in its application to all sports because it employs leg strength, speed, and quickness. It also can be a source of problems if you do not progress into it properly, as described in chapter 3.

Starting Position

Begin by standing at the edge of the elevated platform with the front of the feet just over the edge. Keep the knees slightly bent and the arms relaxed at the sides. The purpose of this position is to facilitate sliding or falling off the edge rather than jumping or stepping off and inadvertently setting a performance rhythm.

Action Sequence

Drop from the elevated surface to the ground (see figures *a* and *b*). While falling, prepare for landing by flexing at the knees and hips. Cock the elbows back and dorsiflex the ankles. Exercise progression begins with repetitions of landing only. Once you have achieved a consistent proper landing position, progress to practicing an immediate takeoff where a jump is initiated upon landing, not after, by thrusting the arms upward and extending the body for as much height as possible (see figure *c*). Maximal intensity and effort are required to produce optimal force while keeping ground contact time to a minimum. Plenty of rest between maximal efforts is necessary as well.

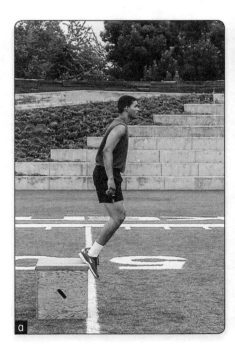
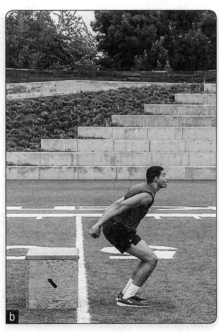
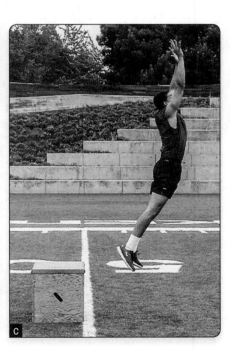

DEPTH LEAP

Introduction

This exercise provides more of an elastic-reactive execution than the normal countermove leap.

Starting Position

Using a stable box or platform at knee-to-hip height, begin by standing at the edge of the elevated platform with the front of the feet just over the edge. Keep the knees slightly bent and the arms relaxed at the sides. The purpose of this position is to facilitate sliding or falling off the edge rather than jumping or stepping off and inadvertently setting a performance rhythm.

Action Sequence

Drop or fall from the elevated surface (see figure *a*), land in takeoff position (see figure *b*), and initiate takeoff immediately upon touchdown (see figures *c-e*). The leap is performed by gaining distance and height outward. The leap is a single, intense effort; therefore, it is helpful to have a pit of sand or foam to cushion the landing (see figure *f*).

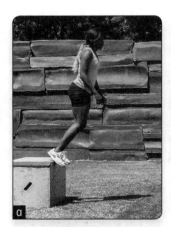
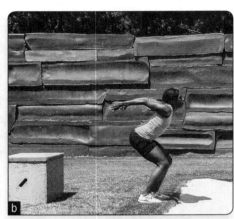
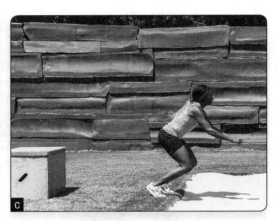
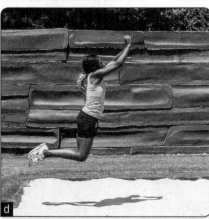
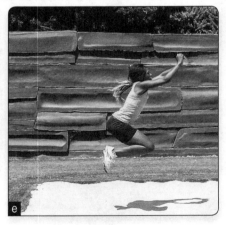
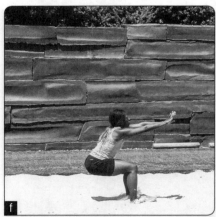

50

DEPTH JUMP LEAP

Introduction

This exercise requires two boxes or benches, one 12 to 16 inches (30 to 40 cm) high and the other 22 to 26 inches (56 to 66 cm) high. Use a resilient landing surface such as grass or a thin mat. This exercise applies to weightlifting, basketball, volleyball, ski jumping, and platform diving.

Starting Position

Stand on the lower box with the arms at the sides; the feet should be together and slightly off the edge as in the depth jump. Place the higher box approximately 2 or 3 feet (60 to 90 cm) in front of and facing you.

Action Sequence

Begin by dropping off the lower box as in depth jumping and landing on both feet (see figures *a* and *b*). Immediately jump onto the higher box, landing on both feet (or on one foot if you are advanced) (see figure *c*), and drive upward and forward as intensely as possible, using the arms and a full extension of the body (see figure *d*). Complete the motion by landing on the ground with both feet and legs flexed to cushion the impact (see figure *e*). Concentrate on a quick, explosive depth jump, overcoming the force of landing, and using the recoil to leap to the higher box. Think of driving hard off the higher box upon landing. As with other shock exercises, you will need rest periods of one to two minutes or more between jumps.

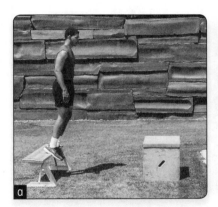
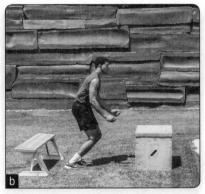
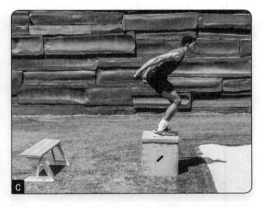

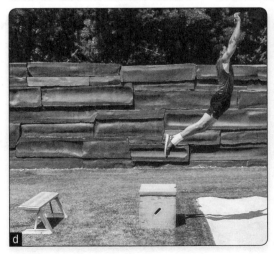
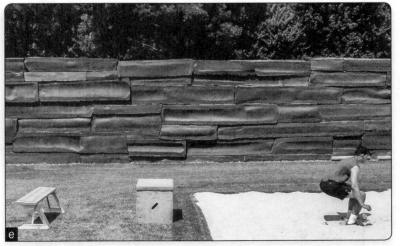

▶ PRANCING

Introduction

As pogo is for jumps, prancing is the beginning progression for bounding. In this exercise it is important to take off and land on both feet simultaneously and to project the hips horizontally.

Starting Position

Assume a standing position with knees slightly bent and the hips tilted forward.

Action Sequence

Upon takeoff, push the hips outward and upward with the knee of one leg recovering forward (see figures a and b). Upon landing, repeat the takeoff with the opposite knee recovering forward (see figure c). The upper-body action is the same as in running. For both feet to land simultaneously, the ankles must remain locked in a toes-up position.

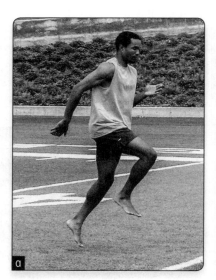 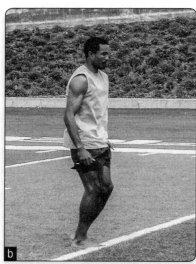 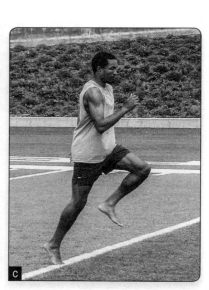

52

▶ GALLOPING

Introduction

Galloping is a rhythmic exercise that fosters good hip projection and back leg push-off. Lead leg mechanics and proper piston and hip extension mechanics are a secondary emphasis.

Starting Position

Assume a standing position with one leg in front of the other.

Action Sequence

Begin by pushing off with the back leg and foot, keeping the ankle locked to emphasize a spring-loaded landing and takeoff (see figure *a*). Continue to keep the same leg behind the hips and project the hips forward while maintaining the opposite leg in a forward position for initial landing and balance within each stride (see figures *b-e*). After executing 6 to 12 repetitions, switch the position of the legs and repeat the sequence. Emphasize hip projection upward and forward with forceful, quick extensions of the back knee and ankle, accompanied by piston-like striding actions of the lead leg.

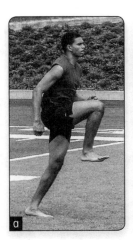 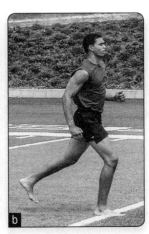 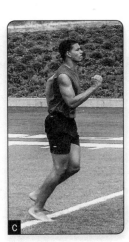 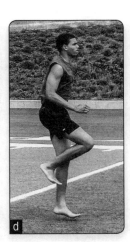 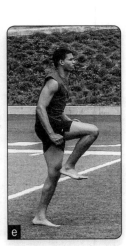

53

Introduction

Skipping is an excellent exercise for working the striding muscles. It reinforces sprinting and jumping mechanics and trains the explosiveness required in the acquisition stages. Fast skipping, or sprinter's skip, as we often refer to it, should resemble high-level acceleration mechanics, maximizing the knee drive of the swing leg and the hip extension from the stance leg. The elbow action is exactly that of acceleration.

Starting Position

Assume a relaxed standing position with one leg slightly forward.

Action Sequence

Begin this sequence with a very dynamic thrust of the swing leg back down onto the ground. As you do, drive the lead-leg toes up, scrape the bottom of the foot from the ground (the hop portion), and drive the knee forward and upward, finishing with the heel up under the hamstring (see figures a-e). Maintain close contact with the ground and emphasize hip projection forward. Do not emphasize stride distances; rather, maximize hip propulsion and thigh extension, recovery, and frequency.

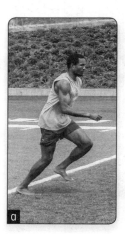 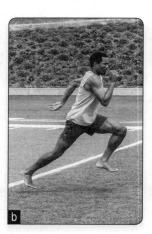 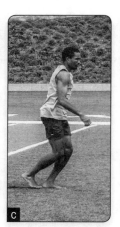 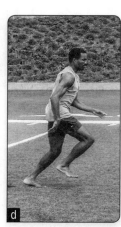 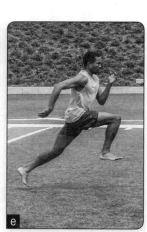

54

POWER SKIPPING

Introduction

Skipping is an excellent exercise for working the striding muscles; it reinforces sprinting and jumping mechanics and trains the explosiveness required in the acquisition stages. Perform all skipping by executing a step-hop pattern of right-right-step to left-left-step to right-right-step, and so on.

Starting Position

Assume a relaxed standing position with one leg slightly forward.

Action Sequence

Drive off the back leg, initiating a short, skipping step; then, with the opposite leg, thrust the toe and knee up (see figure a). Upon landing, repeat the action with the opposite leg (see figures b-d). Obtain as much height and explosive power as possible after each short step. Drive the knee up hard and fast to transfer force from the maximal extension of the support leg. Block with the arms, concentrating on body lift and hang time while minimizing ground contact.

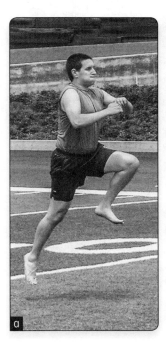
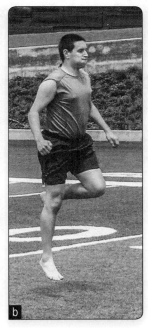
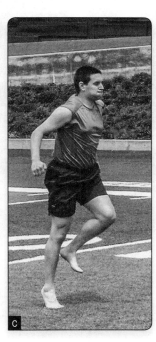
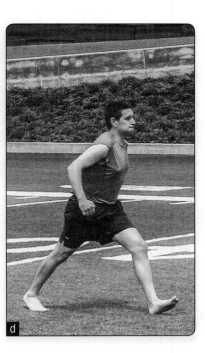

55

Introduction

Skipping is an excellent exercise for working the striding muscles; it reinforces sprinting and jumping mechanics and trains the explosiveness required in the acquisition stages. Perform all skipping by executing a step-hop pattern of right-right-step to left-left-step to right-right-step, and so on.

Starting Position

Assume a relaxed standing position with one leg slightly forward.

Action Sequence

Extended skipping involves a long flight time with each hop and step in the sequence. Maintain good stride mechanics in the step phase while the hop foot covers as much distance as possible to accompany the maximal horizontal knee drive and lead-foot pawing action (see figures *a-e*). The timing and rhythm of extended skipping are similar to those of the triple jump.

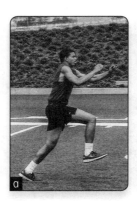
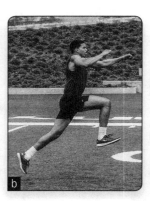
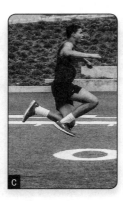
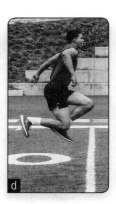
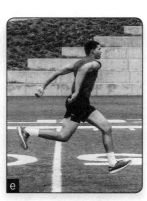

56

▶ ANKLE FLIP

Introduction

Because the ankle flip is performed from one leg onto the other, it is the next level in the progression toward bounding. The ankle flip emphasizes forward hip projection through full extension of the hip and knee.

Starting Position

Assume a relaxed upright stance with one foot forward.

Action Sequence

Begin by pushing the hips forward and outward from the lead foot and leg (see figure *a*). With minimal knee flexion and the ankle locked, land on the opposite foot and quickly extend from that position so the hips remain in a forward thrusting sequence with the ankle always projecting from slightly behind (see figures *b* and *c*). Landing and maximizing ground reaction forces from upward down into or onto the ground are a primary emphasis of this preliminary bounding exercise.

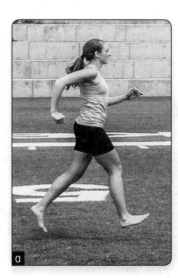
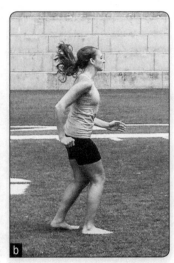
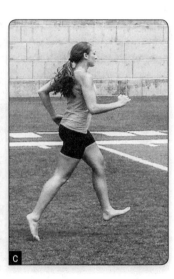

57

Introduction

This exercise can be performed on flat ground or with angled boxes or a similar incline. It emphasizes using the adductors and abductors of the thighs as well as the stabilizing muscles of the knees and ankles. The lateral bound is excellent training for most sports, especially skating, hockey, Nordic skiing, tennis, basketball, and baseball.

Starting Position

Assume a semisquat position that is perpendicular to the destination. If using an angled box or incline, place it approximately one long step away and at the side.

Action Sequence

Emphasizing distance and horizontal trajectory, allow the lead leg to do a countermovement jump inward, shifting the weight to the outside leg for an immediate push-off and extension while the lead shoulder and knee dip and drive for distance (see figures *a* and *b*). The lead foot will land first with the trail foot following to balance the landing (see figure *c*). Perform this exercise using the progressions detailed in chapter 3: single response, multiple response with pause, and multiple response. For single response, use maximal explosion and resetting each time for optimal feedback about your performance, and emphasize using the thigh and groin muscles as well as the hips and low back.

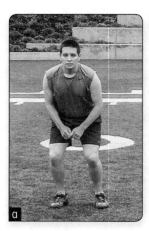
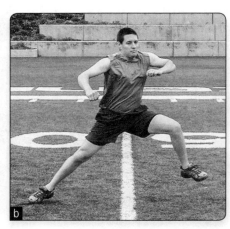
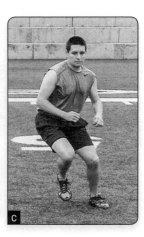

58

▶ SINGLE-LEG STAIR BOUND

Introduction

This exercise emphasizes decreasing the impact of landing on an elevated surface while attending to the mechanics needed for optimal execution. Closed stairs, those having facing panels (e.g., stadium steps, not bleachers), are necessary to ensure that the lead foot does not catch underneath.

Starting Position

Balance on one leg on the second step from the bottom, with the opposite leg poised slightly behind and above the step adjacently below.

Action Sequence

Come off the top foot and drop down to the step below on the opposite foot (see figures *a* and *b*). When the back foot contacts the lower step, immediately explode and push off, simultaneously driving the original lead knee upward and onto a step or two above the starting step (see figures *c* and *d*). This sequence of right leg, drop to left, bound up onto right, galloping continues for an allotted number of repetitions. Then repeat by switching the lead and push-off legs (e.g., left, drop to right, bound to left) and performing the same number of repetitions to complete a set.

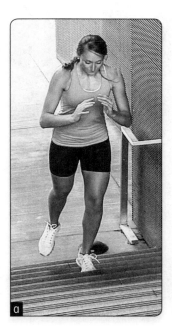 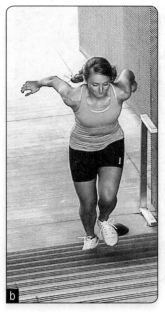 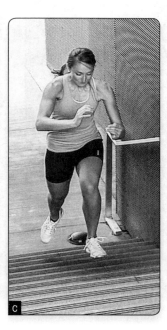 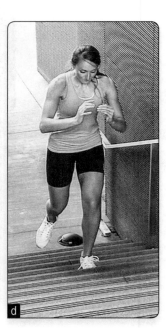

▶ DOUBLE-LEG INCLINE BOUND

Introduction

Perform this exercise on closed stairs, stadium steps, or a sloped hill. Working up the incline reduces the impact of landing forces and places greater emphasis on extension and takeoff forces.

Starting Position

Assume a relaxed semisquat stance on the front portion of the step. Relax the arms and hold them slightly behind the body in preparation for blocking.

Action Sequence

Like many others, this exercise has a progression. Perform the single-response mode on stairs or a hill. Do a countermovement jump into full extension and explosion forward and upward into the incline, followed by flexion into proper, full-foot landings with upright posture (see figures *a-c*). Reset between repetitions. Multiple-response bounds are best performed on steps. From the ready position, drop back onto the previous step to initiate movement. During the drop, maintain a posture that allows hip projection upward and forward. With as rapid a takeoff as possible, bound up as many steps as good landing technique will allow, ready to drop and take off again.

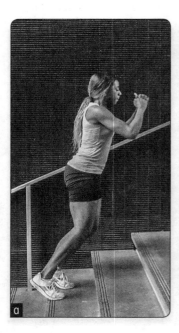
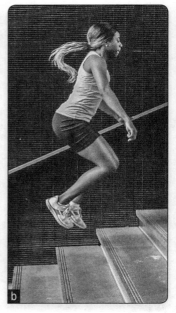
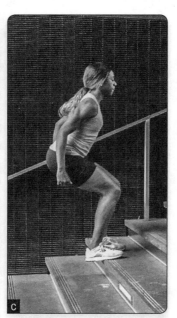

▶ LATERAL STAIR BOUND

Introduction

This exercise is the progressive combination of a multiple-response version of the lateral bound on the decreased landing impact of elevated surfaces. Like the single-leg stair bound, this exercise uses the dropping back of one step and an explosive sideways bounding action up several more.

Starting Position

Begin in a semisquat stance with shoulders perpendicular to the stairs and the weight on the upstairs leg.

Action Sequence

In the same manner as the other stair bound exercises, keep the weight shifted into the steps, drop back one step with the downside leg, and, with immediate extension of that leg and knee, drive off the upside leg and quickly bound upward and inward two or three steps (see figures *a-c*). Continue this drop one, bound two or three up sequence; then repeat facing the opposite direction.

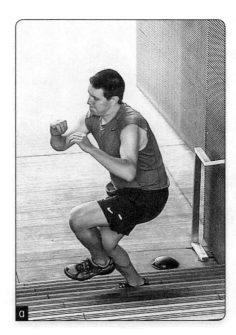 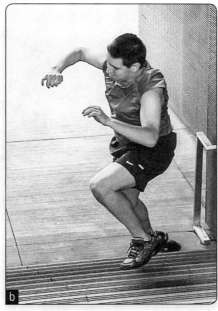 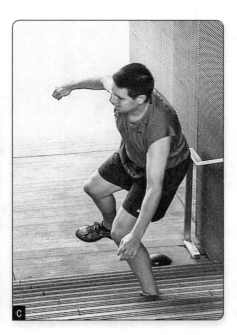

ALTERNATE-LEG STAIR BOUND

Introduction

This exercise is next in the progression of exercises addressing horizontal hip projection. It involves alternate-leg landings of decreased impact using an incline surface such as a hill or enclosed stairs.

Starting Position

Assume a comfortable stance with one foot slightly ahead of the other to initiate a step; the arms should be relaxed and at the sides. Variations on a stationary start are walking and running starts, which improve performance efficiency.

Action Sequence

Begin by running up the steps, with maximal extension of the support leg and maximal knee drive of the swing leg, forward and into the stairs (see figures *a-d*). Maintain a toes-up, heels-up posture for quick takeoffs and explosiveness, and refrain from overstriding and lengthy time on each step.

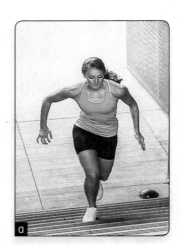
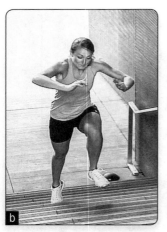
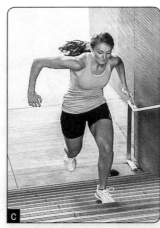
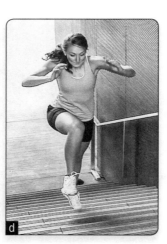

▶ ALTERNATE-LEG BOUND

Introduction

This exercise is the prime exercise for developing explosive leg and hip power. Alternating the legs works the flexor and extensor muscles of the thighs and hips and enhances running, sprinting, and jumping actions.

Starting Position

Assume a comfortable stance with one foot slightly ahead of the other to initiate a step; the arms should be relaxed and at the sides. Variations on a stationary start are walking and running starts, which improve performance efficiency. Other variations include alternating the landings (e.g., right-right-left, left-left-right, right-right-left-left) to emphasize the acceleration and reacceleration of the stride mechanics.

Action Sequence

Begin by pushing off with the back leg and driving the knee forward and upward to gain as much height and distance as possible before landing (see figures *a-e*). Repeat the sequence (driving with the other leg) upon landing. Keep the ankle locked in dorsiflexion and the heel up under the hips to reduce ground contact time and promote efficient hip projection on the subsequent takeoff. Either block with the arms in a contralateral motion, as in normal running, or execute a double-arm swing.

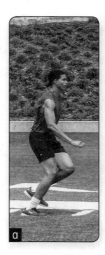
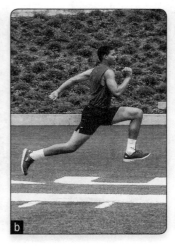
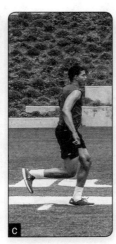
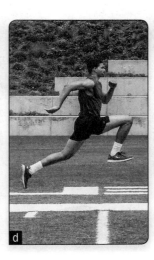
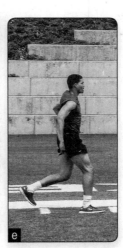

63

Introduction

This exercise introduces a variation of the normal bounding pattern that aids in power cutting maneuvers (lateral changes of direction by planting the outside foot). It enhances the ability to gain distance at angles as well as forward.

Starting Position

Assume a comfortable stance with one foot slightly ahead of the other to initiate a step; the arms should be relaxed and at the sides. Variations on a stationary start are walking and running starts, which improve performance efficiency.

Action Sequence

Begin by pushing off with the back leg, and then drive the knee forward and upward to gain as much height and distance as possible before landing (see figures *a-c*). Repeat the sequence (driving with the other leg) upon landing. Keep the ankle locked in dorsiflexion and the heel up under the hips to reduce ground contact time and promote efficient hip projection on the subsequent takeoff. Either block with the arms in a contralateral motion, as in normal running, or execute a double-arm swing. As you progress in skill, increase the distance from side to side as well as forward upon landing.

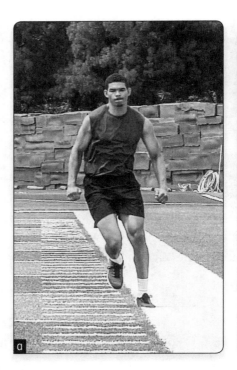
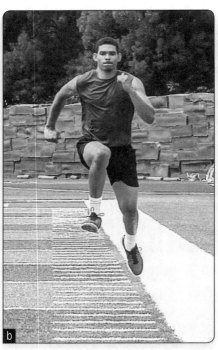
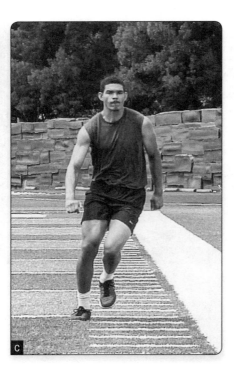

64

BOX SKIP

Introduction

This exercise requires two to four boxes 8 to 24 inches (20 to 60 cm) high. This is an advanced shock-method exercise for elite practitioners involved in jumping events such as track and field, basketball, and volleyball.

Starting Position

Place the boxes in any order of height about 6 to 10 feet (1.8 to 3 m) apart. Facing the first box from about two steps away, assume an upright stance with one leg slightly behind the other. The arms should be relaxed at the sides.

Action Sequence

Drive off the back leg and attempt to gain as much height with the hips as possible. Block with the arms and drive the knee upward to assist in the explosive extension of the push-off leg (see figures *a* and *b*). Immediately upon landing on a box, drive the other leg forward and upward to gain maximal height and distance (see figures *c-e*). Use momentum from this action to leap onto the ground between the first and second boxes with the same leg as the one that landed on the first box; then step to the next box (i.e., skip). Continue this skip action sequence over the remaining boxes. Concentrate on push-off and knee drive with quickness and maximal force to maximize liftoff and hang time.

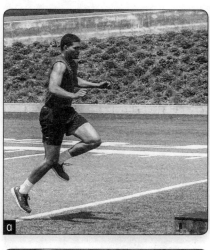
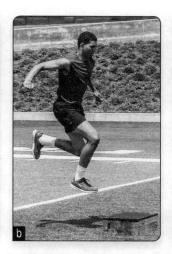
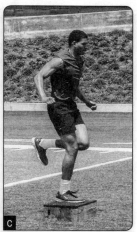

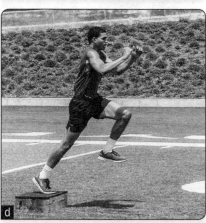
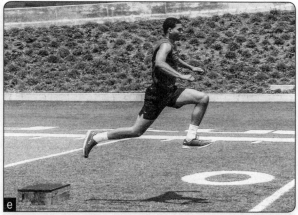

65

BOX BOUND

Introduction

Using two to four boxes 8 to 24 inches (20 to 60 cm) high, as in the box skip exercise, places more resistive overloads on the specific sprinting and jumping musculature. Because this exercise is of shock intensity, it is reserved for athletes in advanced stages of training who are highly competent and have high training maturity. This is why it appears last in this segment's continuum of exercises.

Starting Position

Assume a comfortable stance two or three steps in front of a series of boxes spaced according to your abilities as well as technique. Place one foot slightly ahead of the other to initiate a step; the arms should be relaxed and at the sides.

Action Sequence

Begin by pushing off with the back leg and driving the knee forward and upward to gain as much height and distance as possible before landing (see figures *a* and *b*). Repeat the sequence (driving with the other leg) upon landing as in the alternate-leg bound except that you take every other step from a box (see figures *c-e*). Emphasize landing and foot placement to maintain an erect torso and allow immediate forward hip projection. Eliminate landing positions that foster overstriding or pulling the hips over and off the box.

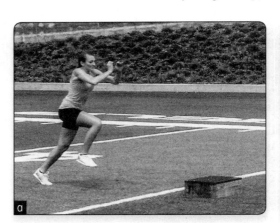
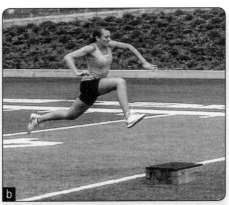
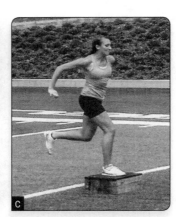
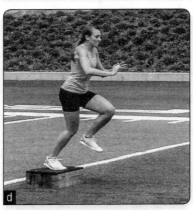
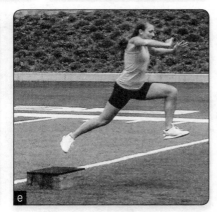

DOUBLE-LEG HOP

Introduction

The hop exercises in this section are presented in a progression. In the early stages, work on developing consistent, proper takeoff and landing techniques. Cones or small hurdles can help.

Starting Position

Assume a relaxed standing position with the knees slightly bent and the arms at the sides. Stand directly in front of a series of three to five hurdles spaced approximately 3 feet (1 m) apart.

Action Sequence

Using a quick countermovement jump, extend the hips for vertical height (see figures *a* and *b*). At full extension, tuck the toes, knees, and heels upward in a cycling motion to clear the hurdle (see figure *c*). Maintain your posture and upright position by blocking with the arms. For single response, upon clearing the first hurdle, land with full-foot contact and give at the knees and hips (see figure *d*). After sticking this landing, pause, and then reset the body position, stance, and relationship to the next hurdle. Then execute the next hop. This reset allows for a reeducation of landing and takeoff technique. Perform this exercise using the progressions detailed in chapter 3: single response, multiple response with pause, and multiple response.

For multiple response, how well you land dictates how well you take off. Execute these hops by pausing for a brief moment, in the best landing position possible, and then perform the next takeoff without resetting the lower or upper body.

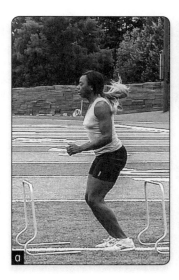
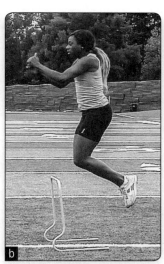
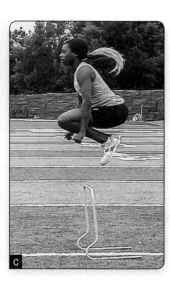
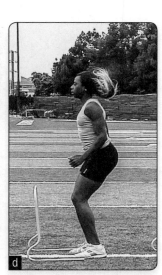

67

▶ DOUBLE-LEG SPEED HOP

Introduction

This exercise builds speed and power in the leg and hip muscles. It is useful for developing explosiveness and specifically applies to the mechanics of speed work required in running.

Starting Position

Assume a relaxed standing position with the knees slightly bent and the arms at the sides. Stand directly in front of a series of three to five hurdles spaced approximately 3 feet (1 m) apart.

Action Sequence

Using a quick countermovement jump, extend the hips for vertical height. At full extension, tuck the toes, knees, and heels upward in a cycling motion to clear the hurdle. Maintain your posture and upright position by blocking with the arms. Upon each landing, take off quickly upward with the same cycling action of the legs. Execute the action sequence as rapidly as possible. Work for height and distance, but not at the expense of repetition rate.

▶ INCREMENTAL VERTICAL HOP

Introduction

This exercise requires elastic tubing or a rope approximately 15 feet (5 m) long. Attach one end to a wall or pole at eye level and the other end to a semireleasable object at ground level. This exercise is excellent for all activities because it enhances stability during explosive cycling action.

Starting Position

With feet together, assume a relaxed position facing the wall or pole and immediately to the side of the lower end of the rope or tubing. Prepare the arms for blocking to provide lift.

Action Sequence

Hopping back and forth over the tubing, advance up the tubing as high as possible (see figures a-d). Bring the knees forward and upward toward the chest while tucking the feet underneath the hips. Continue up the tubing as far as possible, thus completing the set.

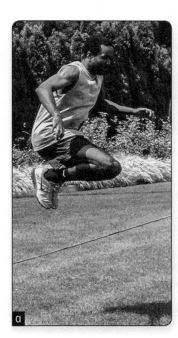 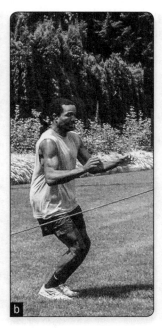 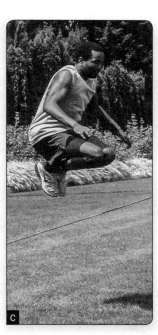 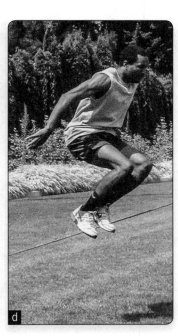

69

Introduction

This exercise requires two cones approximately 18 to 26 inches (46 to 66 cm) high. The movement specifically enhances explosive lateral power throughout the legs and hips. This exercise is useful for all activities employing lateral movement.

Starting Position

Set both cones side by side approximately 2 feet (60 cm) apart; increase the distance progressively as performance improves. Assume a relaxed upright stance to the outside of one cone (see figure a). Keep the feet together and pointing straight ahead, and cock the arms to be ready to provide lift and aid in balance.

Action Sequence

With both feet, take off sideways over the first cone (see figures b-d) and then the second one. Without hesitating, change direction by jumping back over the second cone and then the first one. Continue this back-and-forth sequence. Block with the arms in an upward thrusting motion to aid in lift and maintain your posture.

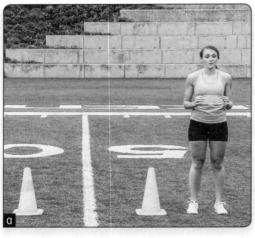
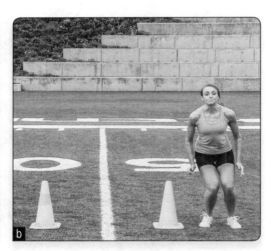
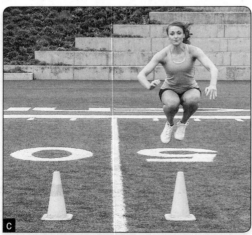
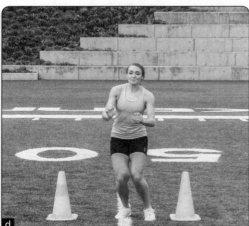

70

SIDE HOP-SPRINT

Introduction

This exercise requires a bag, low bench, tackling dummy, or similar object to hop over. Combining a series of hops with a full sprint for a short, accelerated distance, this exercise enhances the coordination needed for rapidly changing direction. It applies to tennis, basketball, baseball, football, and many other sports that require changes of direction.

Starting Position

Stand on one side of the bag with feet together and pointing straight ahead. An advanced progression would be to stand with your back to the bag and the toes pointing directly away from it.

Action Sequence

Begin by hopping sideways back and forth over the bag for a designated number of repetitions (approximately six) (see figures *a-d*). Execute the hops as rapidly and efficiently as possible. The primary objective of the exercise is to work on the rate of execution, not the height of the hops. Keep the trunk and hips centered over the bag, because posture is of prime importance to optimal execution. Anticipate the landing on the last repetition; land in a sprint starting posture and accelerate forward past a designated finish line (see figure *e*). Several participants using several bags can race; the participant completing the designated number of hops first would have an advantage in finishing first.

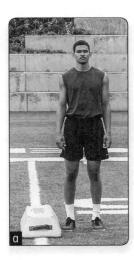
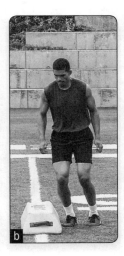
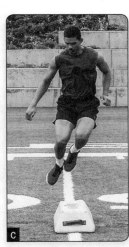
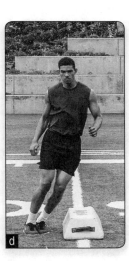
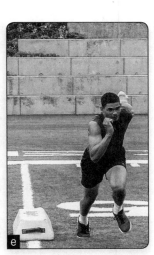

71

Introduction

This exercise is best performed on a multiple-angle box or similar apparatus, which must be securely attached to the ground so it does not move or slip during the hops. Angle hops improve balance and lateral movement. This exercise is useful for alpine skiing, tennis, American football, and gymnastics, as well as other sports.

Starting Position

Stand in a relaxed position on one angled surface of the box.

Action Sequence

Hop laterally from one side of the box to the next sequentially, emphasizing a rapid side-to-side and forward motion (see figures *a-c*). At the apex of the hop, the knees are brought up toward the body (see figure *d*). Once skill has improved, progress to more distinct angles. Block with the arms for balance.

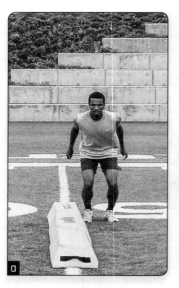
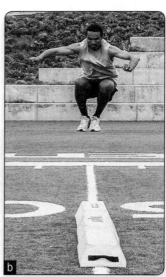
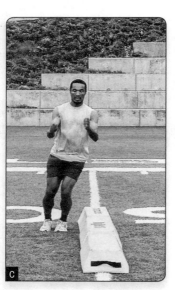
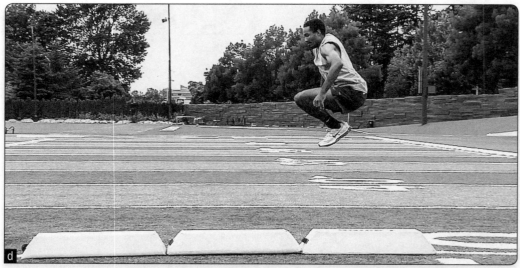

▶ SINGLE-LEG POGO

Introduction

This exercise enhances landing and takeoff mechanics from the ankle through the hip. This beginning single-leg exercise helps train or rehabilitate sprinting posture and ground negotiation. This exercise is crucial for training directing sprinting ground reaction forces downward into the ground from an erect position directly above the contact point, as mentioned in earlier chapters.

Starting Position

Stand tall with one leg flexed at the hip, the ankle lifted and locked, and the toes up. The knee should be held above the level of the hip, with the heel in front of the support knee.

Action Sequence

Flex and then extend the support leg upward and forward (see figures *a* and *b*). Land each time on the full foot, with the shin and body weight over the instep (see figure *c*). Each landing and takeoff should be felt high in the upper leg and hip, not around the knee (which indicates landing too much on the toes). Variations from barefoot are landings on targets (plates) to create full-foot, stabilized landings. Variations of the forward pogo action are lateral takeoffs and landings both to the inside and outside of each leg. If posture begins to falter, the repetitions are too high or the distance of travel is too far.

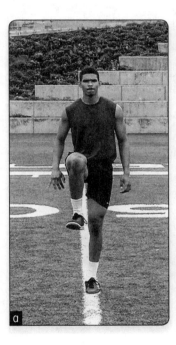
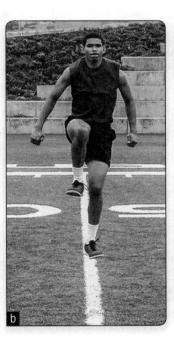
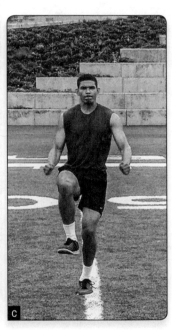

73

Introduction

This exercise has prime value in all sprinting and single-leg jumping activities. It is also excellent for determining the ability to handle the posture, balance, stability, and flexibility of single-leg work.

Starting Position

Adopt an upright stance with knees slightly bent, chest out, and shoulders back. Lift one leg by pulling the heel upward at hip level and the heel up underneath the hamstring. As mentioned, this position is very important for training postural-integrity sprint mechanics.

Action Sequence

Using a quick countermovement jump, extend the hips for vertical height (see figures *a-c*). At full extension, tuck the toes and heel of the takeoff leg upward as if backed up against a wall, thereby needing to slide the heels up. The knee rises upward and forward attempting to match the position of the other knee. Maintain your posture and upright position by blocking with the arms. Perform all the repetitions with one leg; then switch to the other. Perform this exercise using the progressions detailed in chapter 3: single response, multiple response with pause, and multiple response.

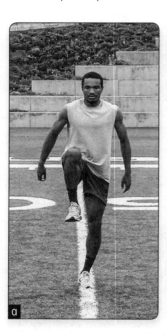 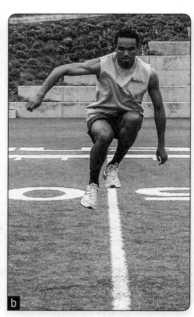 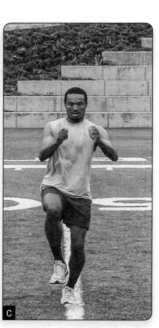

SINGLE-LEG HOP

Introduction

The double-leg hop technique applies to advancing into hopping in its most definitive form, with a single leg. Evaluation of optimal posture, balance, stability, and flexibility is even more important with one-leg landings and takeoffs over a row of small cones or minihurdles.

Starting Position

Assume a relaxed standing position with the knees slightly bent and the arms at the sides. Completely balance on one leg while keeping the other leg in a flexed position with the toes up, the knee in front of the body at hip level, and the heel up underneath the hamstring (see figure *a*).

Action Sequence

Using the countermoving effects of the swing leg for lift and drive, and at full extension, tuck the toes, knees, and heels upward in a cycling motion to clear the cones or minihurdles (see figures *b-d*). Maintain your posture and upright position by blocking with the arms. Upon each landing, take off quickly upward again with the same cycling action of the legs. Execute the action sequence as rapidly as possible. Work for height and distance, but not at the expense of repetition rate.

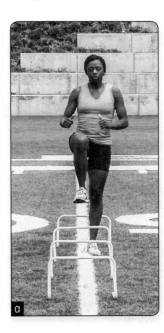
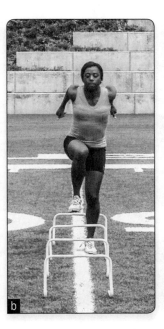
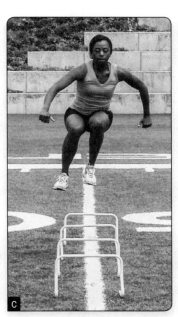
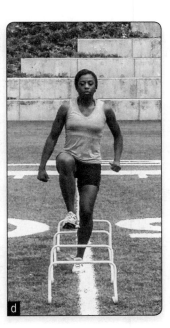

75

SINGLE-LEG SPEED HOP

Introduction

This multiple-response version of true hopping is the ultimate exercise for developing the explosive, reactive, and cyclic action of sprinting. The skill requirements are the same as for the single-leg hop.

Starting Position

Assume a relaxed standing position with the knees slightly bent and the arms at the sides. Completely balance on one leg while keeping the other leg in a flexed position with the toes up, the knee in front of the body at hip level, and the heel up underneath the hamstring.

Action Sequence

Use the multiple-response action of rapid yet fully explosive cyclic action for height and distance. Using a quick countermovement jump, extend the hips for vertical height, and at full extension, tuck the toes, knees, and heels upward in a cycling motion. Maintain your posture and upright position by blocking with the arms. Upon each landing, take off quickly upward again with the same cycling action of the stance leg. Execute the action sequence as rapidly as possible. Display the locked ankle, heel up, and fast recovering action necessary for optimal execution.

SINGLE-LEG DIAGONAL HOP

Introduction

This exercise is slightly higher in stress load than the previous straight-ahead single-leg hop progression because of the lateral stability necessary for performing these takeoffs and landings.

Starting Position

Assume a relaxed standing position to one side of a series of small (6-12 in.) cones or collapsible hurdles, with the knees slightly bent and the arms at the sides. Completely balance on one leg while keeping the other leg in a flexed position with the toes up, the knee in front of the body at hip level, and the heel up underneath the hamstring (see figure *a*).

Action Sequence

Upon takeoff, project the hips at a 45-degree angle inside or outside the takeoff point for a diagonal path, forward down the cone line (see figures *b-d*). Progress by performing the exercise to the outside, then inside, and finally, crossing back and forth.

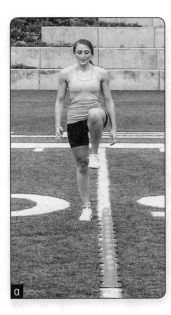
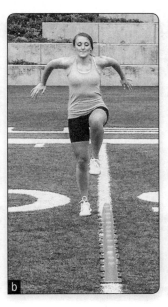
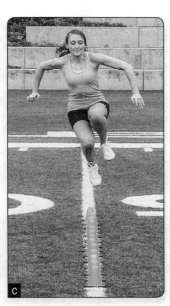
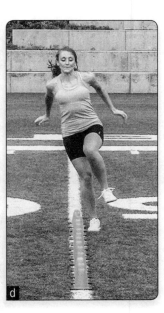

SINGLE-LEG LATERAL HOP

Introduction

This is an excellent exercise for training lateral movement and improving the execution of speed and power cutting in athletic movements.

Starting Position

Assume a relaxed standing position with the knees slightly bent and the arms relaxed to the side of a row of small cones or imaginary hurdles placed perpendicular to the stance. Completely balance on one leg while keeping the other leg in a flexed position with the toes up, the knee in front of the body at hip level, and the heel up underneath the hamstring (see figure *a*).

Action Sequence

Upon takeoff, project the hips directly to the side of the takeoff point. Then execute the vertical lift and pistonlike leg action over cones or imaginary minihurdles. The key is to keep upright postural control while flexing the hopping leg upward at the hip rather than backward at the knee (see figures *b-d*). Progress by performing the exercise to the outside, to the inside, or back and forth.

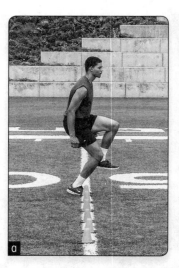
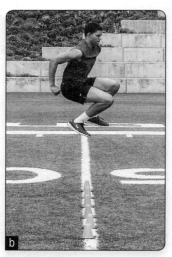
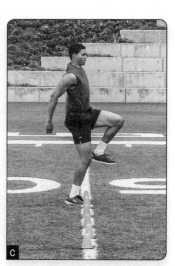
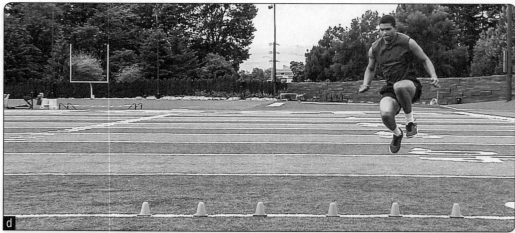

78

DECLINE HOP

Introduction

Use a grassy hill of about 1 to 3 degrees of inclination. (*Note:* Do not attempt this exercise on steps, bleachers, or a wet, slick surface.) This exercise develops elastic reactivity in the lower body through increased shock on the musculature and increased downward speed.

Starting Position

Assume a quarter-squat stance at the top of the hill with the body facing down the fall line.

Action Sequence

Execute this movement the same as all other forward hopping movements. Execute the hops by gaining vertical height and cycling the feet up over imaginary knee-high hurdles that are placed in a line down the incline runway. (see figures *a-c*). Performing this hop on the decline requires even greater emphasis on repetition rate and movement speed, so this exercise is suggested only after mastering all of the previous hop exercises.

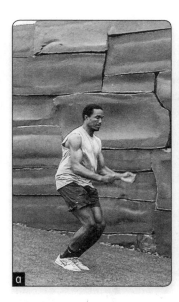
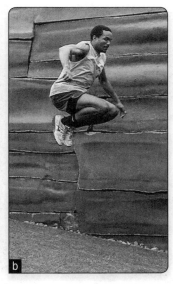
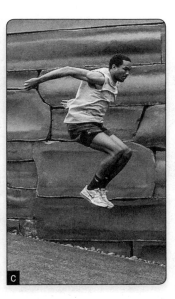

INCLINE RICOCHET

Introduction

This exercise requires a set of stairs or stadium steps. The stairs must be solid, with no openings in which toes and feet may become entrapped. This exercise trains reflexive quickness in more of an unloaded, or overspeed, manner. It is well suited for all sports involving fast footwork.

Starting Position

Stand at the bottom of the steps facing them in a relaxed upright position with feet together and arms to the sides and cocked at the elbows.

Action Sequence

Rapidly move up every step at the highest rate possible without tripping (see figures *a-c*). Use the arms for balance, keeping the thumbs up, and also for assisting in explosion from step to step. Quickness is most important in this exercise, so focus on relaxation. Anticipate hopping or stepping rapidly to each succeeding step. Think of being light on the feet. Variations of the ricochet include angling to the right or left of the steps or facing completely sideways. The ricochet can be done with feet together, in carioca step fashion, with a four-step sequence, or on one leg if you are advanced.

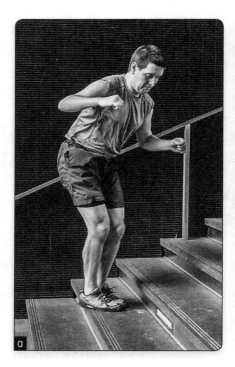
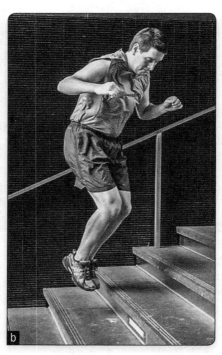
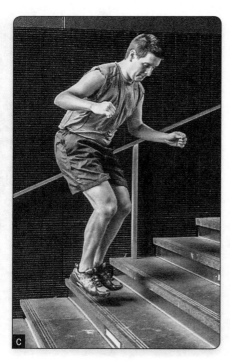

PART III

Plyometric Programming

Complex Training

Complex training is the coupling of strength and speed, or the incorporating of training loads, speeds, and styles in the quest for athletic power. Complex training requires exercises that are biomechanical and athletically specific (especially in terms of velocities) to the endeavors of the athlete's sport. Olympic-style lifts that employ the entire body across multiple joints and use highly synchronized loads and speeds are very applicable to the biomechanics of many sports and athletic activities. This training mode should be performed early in the workout when dynamic work is optimal, prior to any heavily loaded, slow, or single-joint isolation exercises. This provides greater work intensity and velocity and the inclusion of multijoint combinations (Ebben and Blackard 1997). This chapter offers several definitions and examples of both complex and combination training and explains their applications to program design.

Definitions of complex training have existed for many years. In 1966 Verkhoshansky described it as a complex of exercises united according to the principle that basic exercises for the development of reactive ability via heightened excitability of the CNS by exercise requiring great power. In 1986 Fleck and Kontor described it as a series of exercises performed in succession designed to increase the ability to produce power quickly. Chu (1996) suggested the definition of a workout system that combines strength work and speed work for an optimal training effect. Ebben and Blackard (1997) explained complex training as a training system that alternates biomechanically similar high-load weight training and plyometric exercises, set for set, within the same workout. They considered it a convenient and optimal training strategy for the development of sport-specific athletic power. The loads in the weight training sets complement those in the ensuing elastic–reactive exercise sets, thereby optimizing neuromuscular adaptations.

Our definition of complex training is training that involves alternating sets of two exercise styles by set (e.g., a set of one exercise followed by a set of another). Combination training, on the other hand, we define as the alternating of two exercise styles within a single set, or by rep. For example, we consider a set of three repetitions of the clean and jerk to be combination training (clean and jerk). An athlete performs one clean repetition, followed by the jerk repetition, then repeats this sequence twice more. Had the athlete completed all three clean repetitions followed by the three jerk repetitions, this would be complex training (clean, then jerk) (Gambetta and Radcliffe 1989).

Complex training methods can also involve combining two exercises that are similar in movement pattern and yet different in terms of absolute or relative strength (speed is not a factor), and those of elastic (speed and rebound ability). Ebben and Blackard (1997) considered two biomechanically similar exercises to be a complex pair; including a third similar exercise creates a complex triad.

For further definitions of these strength terms, refer to chapter 2. Complexes of absolute strength and elastic strength (weights and plyometrics) that we have found to be effective are squatting then jumping, pressing then passing, pulling then tossing or throwing, and lunging then bounding or skipping.

Following are examples of sequences that combine strength and speed exercises.

Barbell Back Squat Then Squat Jump × 4

Perform a set of four repetitions of the barbell back squat followed immediately by a set of four squat jumps; then rest. Increase the weight of the barbell; then repeat the sequence for three more sets. You may eventually perform the squat jumps with a light weight, such as a 25-pound (or 10 kg) sandbag. In the beginning use only body weight.

Incline Press or Bench Press Then Medicine Ball Chest Pass (for height) × 5

Perform a set of five repetitions of the incline press followed immediately by five repetitions of the medicine ball chest pass with a 7- to 15-pound (3 to 7 kg) medicine ball; then rest. Increase the weight on the barbell if necessary to intensify the repetitions, and repeat the sequence. Do not increase the weight of the medicine ball.

HOW COMPLEX TRAINING WORKS

The rationale for complex training is relatively simple. Practitioners claim that complex training offers the following benefits:

- Better use of time within the workout session
- Better use of floor and work space within the training area
- More efficient use of equipment (e.g., barbells, dumbbells, medicine balls)
- Increase in quality training volume (keeping a power perspective to the sets and reps)
- Increase in the variations of workout and training cycles
- Increase in metabolic work capacity

Chapter 1 addressed the concepts of strength work as well as the aspects of rate of force development (RFD). Strength work alone is not as beneficial in this process, especially when comparing time of force for a heavy squat to the rate of force in athletic ground contact times. Developing rate of force and the neuromuscular components involved (Type IIx muscle fibers) requires a combination of strength and elastic–reactive work.

On some combined strength and elastic workdays, strength, speed, and elastic complexes provide an efficient use of time and the facility. Complex training in this way can result in greater neuromuscular recruitment and subsequent improvements in RFD. The concept is that, when matching pairs of biomechanically similar exercises, the resistance exercise stimulates the central nervous system (CNS) into greater action, recruiting more Type IIx fibers for the explosive exercise.

Many researchers and practitioners describe the physiological rationale for complexing as follows:

- The precontraction of antagonistic muscles counters the inhibitory neural mechanisms in the agonists (Fees 1997).
- Combination programs may produce superior strength and power performance measurements as observed in weightlifters' power outputs and rate of force development (Harris et al. 2000)
- A wider range of stimuli to the muscle encourages the development of both speed and strength. This is due to an increase in motor neuron excitability (Jones and Lees 2003).
- Increased excitability of the CNS occurs as a result of postactivation potentiation (PAP). Heavy loading induces neural stimulation, which improves muscle twitch force (French et al. 2003).

Participants must work at high intensities during both the strength and the speed portions of the complex. As a result, the volume should be low enough to guard against undue fatigue; limited repetitions of all-out efforts should be performed to ensure these intensities. Complex training may be used from one to three times per week with adequate recovery between sessions (recommendations are for at least 48 and not more than 96 hours).

Experts vary widely in their recommendations for the timing of within-set rest periods (from 30 seconds to 20 minutes). The optimal range for performance improvement seems to be between three and eight minutes. Obviously, given that one of the reasons for the use of complex or combined training sequences is a more efficient use of time, the optimal recommendation for within-set rest periods is from one to four minutes. In a review of the research, Ebben (2002) concluded that four minutes was the preferred time allotment. Comyns and colleagues (2006) found similar benefits in rest interval but also supported the use of individually assigning rest intervals for optimal performance. A review of the research also offered a look at effectiveness. Eleven of 14 studies indicated positive effects of complex training protocols. Two studies offered no evidence of effectiveness, and one revealed negative training effects. The results of a more recent study of complex training effects on power development suggested that the method may not be better than traditional training methods that use either strength training or plyometric training on their own. On the other hand, it did not reveal any decrement. Therefore, because complex training incorporates multiple methods into a single work session, it offers effective variable and efficient training (MacDonald et al. 2013).

The benefits of this training style appear to be organizational, although improvements seem to increase over time with continued training. Significant strength levels and plyometric progressions (along the continuum) should be a requirement for application (Duthie, Young, and Aitken 2002).

Probably most important in the practice of complex training methodologies is understanding the biomechanical requirements of the activities being matched and then working from that point forward in a progressive manner. As depicted in figure 8.1, some of the strength and speed, or strength versus speed, qualities can be combined with biomechanical qualities, direction of force applications, and reactive response modes.

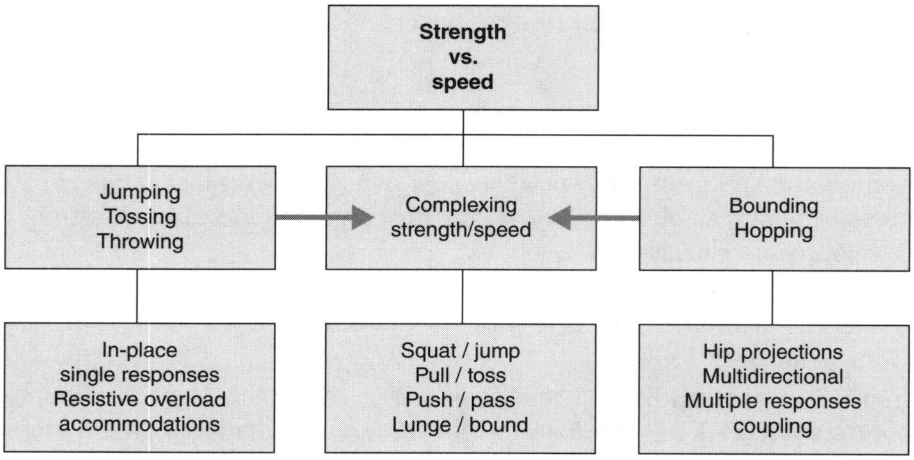

Figure 8.1   Combinations of concepts.

PLANNING COMPLEX TRAINING

As with all forms of training, a model of planned performance protocols, or periodization, is implemented to optimize progressive improvement. Complex training is of greatest value when placed at certain times in training and competitive periods, phases, and cycles. If complex training were to occur prior to working on technical and biological development, it would not be as beneficial. For example, placing a complex of squats and jumps into the training before the athlete has achieved good squat technique at fairly high loads, and before he could execute good jumping techniques of fairly high quality, the complex would have much less value. As explained in earlier chapters, proper planning and progression throughout both the strength training and the plyometric work leads to better performance when it is time to couple the two.

Within the yearly plan of training for performance enhancement, progressions are used in the postseason, off-season, and preseason training periods. Because the specific technical developments can be acquired in the postseason and the off-season, the precompetitive training period is the ideal time to begin plugging in complex training.

EXERCISE METHODOLOGIES

Once we understand the concepts behind what, when, how, and why we are complexing the training methods, the list of possible exercise combinations is vast. However, we must keep in mind that one of the main goals of this process is to optimize training efficiency. Creating a complicated set of exercises just because we can will only slow down or negate some of the positive effects of the methodology. Being in tune with the why of exercise selection is the key. Taking that into account, following are a few of the categories and modes of complex and combination exercises.

Lifting Complexes

Lifting complexes are repetitions of two or more lifting exercise movements within the same set. The following complexes provide a sample of exercises in the pulling, squatting, and pushing categories and show how they interact to aid in movement synchronization.

Pull–Squat

Double- or single-leg good morning; and overhead or back squat, lunge, or step-up

Double- or single-leg deadlift; and overhead or front squat, lunge, or step-up

Clean; and front squat, lunge, or step-up

Snatch; and overhead squat, lunge, or step-up

Squat–Push

Overhead squat or lunge; and press or jerk

Front squat, lunge, or step-up; and press or jerk

Back squat, lunge, or step-up; and press or jerk

Push–Squat

Press from behind or in front; and squat, lunge, or step-up

Jerk from behind or in front; and squat, lunge, or step-up

Pull–Push

Double- or single-leg good morning; and press or jerk from behind

Double- or single-leg deadlift; and press or jerk from the front

Clean; and press or jerk from the front

Snatch; and press or jerk from behind

Pull–Squat–Push or Pull–Push–Squat

Double- or single-leg good morning; press or jerk from behind; and overhead squat, lunge, or step-up

Double- or single-leg deadlift; press or jerk from the front; and overhead squat, lunge, or step-up

Clean; front squat or lunge; and press or jerk

Lifting Combinations

Lifting combinations involve barbells or dumbbells and alternate repetitions of two or more lifting styles within the same set.

Pull–Squat

Double- or single-leg good morning; and overhead or back squat, lunge, or step-up

Double- or single-leg deadlift; and overhead or front squat, lunge, or step-up

Clean; and front squat, lunge, or step-up

Snatch; and overhead squat, lunge, or step-up

Squat–Push

Overhead squat or lunge; and press or jerk

▶ Front squat, lunge, or step-up; and press or jerk

Back squat, lunge, or step-up; and press or jerk

Push–Squat

▶ Press from behind or in front; and squat, lunge, or step-up

Jerk from behind or in front; and squat, lunge, or step-up

Pull–Push

Double- or single-leg good morning; and press or jerk from behind

Double- or single-leg deadlift; and squat, lunge, or step-up from the front

Clean; and press or jerk from the front

Snatch; and press or jerk from behind

Pull–Squat–Push or Pull–Push–Squat

Double- or single-leg good morning; press or jerk from behind; and overhead squat, lunge, or step-up

▶ Double- or single-leg deadlift; press or jerk from the front; and overhead squat, lunge, or step-up

Clean; front squat or lunge; and press or jerk

Snatch; overhead squat or lunge; and press or jerk

Strength and Speed Complexes

In the beginning of this chapter, our definition of complexing focused on the combinations of heavy strength work and dynamic elastic–reactive work. Following are some strength and speed complexes and their exercise modes.

Pull and Toss or Throw

The following movements are biomechanically and dynamically alike:

Clean or snatch pull; and medicine ball toss or throw

Clean or snatch pull; and bar kip-up

Clean or snatch; and medicine ball toss or throw or kip-up

Clean or snatch; and rocket, star, or tuck jump

▶ Split snatch; and split or scissors jump

Squat or Lunge and Jump or Bound

The following movements are biomechanically and dynamically alike:

▶ Overhead, front, or back squat; and squat, rocket, or tuck jump

Overhead, front, or back squat; and double-leg stair bound

Overhead, front, or back lunge; and split, scissors, or stride jump

Overhead, front, or back lunge; and single-leg stair bound or lunge jump

▶ 45-degree or side lunge; and stride jump crossover or diagonal, or lateral (stair) bound

Push and pass

The following movements are biomechanically and dynamically alike:

Push press or jerk (in front or from behind); and squat or squared chest pass

Split jerk (in front or from behind); and staggered heavy bag press punch

Bench or incline press; and medicine ball chest pass or drop push-up (similar angles)

Dumbbell alternating press; and medicine ball wall put (shot style)

▶ Front or back squat; and medicine ball squat chest pass

Pull and Squat or Push and Hop

The following movements are biomechanically and dynamically alike:

Clean, snatch, or squat; and double-leg speed hop

Split snatch, lunge, or split jerk; and single-leg speed hop

45-degree or side lunge, and diagonal or side hop

Pull and Throw

The following movements are biomechanically and dynamically opposite:

▶ Clean, snatch, or high pull; and medicine ball overhead throw forward (kneeling or standing)

Clean, snatch, or high pull; and floor or bar kip-up

The list of types, subtypes, and styles of complex training methodology is long. Those outlined here can be either hugely expanded or meticulously pared down according to training objectives.

We like to use the lifting complexes and combinations for specific warm-up routines with a bar or dumbbells, especially once time gets tight (e.g., during in-season training). The heavier lifting complexes and combinations are especially handy during the preseason and in-season, because time is a factor and optimally coordinated and synchronized lifting and performing is important. We try to take three or four minutes between the loaded strength sets and the dynamic, or elastic, set. When time becomes an issue, such as during in-season training, the time between the strength and speed sets is as follows: a heavy set of few repetitions (two to five) followed by a change of weights (if necessary) for the training partners; then the dynamic, or elastic, set (30 seconds maximum), followed by a change of the weight again; then the third partner goes, and the sequence repeats. We have found this to be a very good use of load, intensity, and time.

Sport-Specific Training

One way to take advantage of explosive training is to tailor exercises to the sport played. Doing so not only motivates athletes because they know that the exercises will help them in their sports, but also gives direction to the individual workouts and progressions. You should not alter the plan to progress from general to specific, from simple to complex, from low to high and shock intensity.

The following plyometric workout programs follow the stress continuum. The first section in each table offers an all-encompassing, basic continuum of exercises to use at the beginning of all plyometric training programs. Sport-specific exercises, known as the sport's desirables, follow. These can accompany the program basics as the athlete progresses through the continuum. Athletes can use any program for the full 12 weeks or any length of time. Athletes and coaches can tailor the time individually or to fit the phasic constraints of the periodized training cycle (see chapter 10). For example, collegiate athletes who are on the quarter system of the academic calendar rarely get a full 12 weeks of training without a break. Therefore, they must step back a week or two and continue to progress with the continuum. The exercise dosage in each column is for spreading over two days within the week. We call these continuum cards for specific sports.

After these sport-specific exercises we present a special feature for beyond basic continuum training—what we call mountains and rivers. These routines, named for particular mountains and rivers based on their use of power, stability, and continual flow toward certain goals, are advanced and appropriate for the competitive phase of training.

Following is a list of sports and activities in no particular order or ranking; these are simply the most common ones we and our colleagues deal with regularly. If your particular sport or activity is not listed here, do not let that deter you. You know your sport or activity well, and with the guidelines in this book and the following examples, you will be able to set up your own continuum card of specific training.

Soccer

Baseball, softball, and cricket

Volleyball

Cycling

Field hockey

Basketball and netball

Rowing

American football

Skiing

Lacrosse

Tennis, racquetball, squash, and handball

Track and field

Olympic weightlifting

Wrestling

Aussie football

12-WEEK CONDITIONING PROGRAMS

Tables 9.1 through 9.21 present comprehensive, progressive plyometric training programs for a variety of sports. The first 12 exercises at the top of each table are called program basics because they are general conditioning exercises for any training program, regardless of the sport. These basic exercises are a lead-in, and they increase in complexity and specificity as the weeks continue.

The first few weeks of each program consist of program basics and, in most cases, only a few sport-specific exercises. We call these sport-specific exercises the desirables. Athletes should perform these exercises on the same days as the program basics exercises. Eventually, some exercises may become technical training, or even the warm-up, but during the 12-week program they are the training itself. Each coach or athlete may add others or replace some with others; they know their sports and activities and can apply the principles discussed. For continuity, we provide 12 exercises for basic training and specific sport work. Numbers represent the number of sets and repetitions (e.g., 2 × 4-6 indicates two sets of four to six repetitions).

As mentioned, athletes should spread the exercises for each week over two days, preferably with one or more days of nonelastic–reactive work between them (refer to the section Rest in chapter 3). They can split the workload by doing half the volume of every exercise on each of the two days. However, in some cases, as in several of the third to eighth weeks, 14 to 18 exercises may be scheduled for the week. What we have found to work well is to split the exercises into two groups, either basics and specifics, or, even better, to split them up to match the style of training for that day. Let's say that on the third week an athlete has the 11 program basics exercises as well as 5 to 10 desirable exercises. On day 1, she does lifting and sprinting as well as the exercises. On day 2, she does just the sprinting and the exercises. In this case, she should choose some program basics exercises that fit either with the lifting (perhaps in complex style), such as pogo, squat jump, box jump, split jump, or star jump, or with the sprinting, such as prancing, galloping, skipping, or ankle flip. We could term this a vertical versus horizontal split in the week's exercises. On the other hand, we have found it useful to split the exercises by complexity or intensity, with the first several basics and desirable exercises on the day that has lifting and running, and the latter exercises of each section on the day with only sprint training.

Table 9.1 Continuum Training for Soccer

Exercise	Page #	Wk 1	Wk 2	Wk 3	Wk 4	Wk 5	Wk 6	Wk 7	Wk 8	Wk 9	Wk 10	Wk 11	Wk 12
PROGRAM BASICS													
Pogo	104	3 × 10	3 × 10	3 × 10	3 × 10								
Squat jump	105	2 × 4-6	3 × 4-6	3 × 6-8									
Medicine ball over and under, medicine ball half and full twist	88, 92, and 93	3 × 3	3 × 4	3 × 5	3 × 6	3 × 6							
Rocket jump and star jump	107 and 108	2 × 4-6	2 × 4-6	3 × 4-6		3 × 4-6							
Split jump and scissors jump	111 and 112	2 × 4-6		3 × 4-6	3 × 6-8	3 × 6-8	3 × 4-6						
Prancing	120	2 × 4-6	2 × 4-6	2 × 4-6	2 × 4-6	2 × 4-6							
Galloping	121	3 × 10	3 × 10	3 × 10	3 × 10	2 × 10	2 × 10	2 × 10	2 × 10	2 × 10	2 × 10	2 × 10	2 × 10
Fast skipping	122	3 × 10	3 × 10	3 × 10	3 × 10	2 × 10	2 × 10	2 × 10	2 × 10	2 × 10	2 × 10	2 × 10	2 × 10
Ankle flip	125	2 × 4-6	3 × 4-6	3 × 4-6	3 × 6-8	3 × 6-8	3 × 6-8	3 × 6-8	3 × 6-8	3 × 6-8	2 × 8-10	2 × 8-10	2 × 8-10
Single-leg stair bound	127		2 × 4-6	2 × 4-6	3 × 6-8		2 × 8-10	2 × 8-10		2 × 8-10			
Lateral bound (single response)	126			2 × 6-8	3 × 6-8	3 × 8-10	3 × 8-12		3 × 10-12				
Alternate-leg stair bound	130		2 × 6-8	3 × 6-8	3 × 8-10	3 × 8-12	3 × 8-12	3 × 8-12					
DESIRABLES													
Incline ricochet	148			3 × 8-12	3 × 8-12	3 × 8-12		3 × 8-12	3 × 8-12				
Knee-tuck jump	110			3 × 4-6	3 × 4-6	3 × 4-6	3 × 4-6	3 × 4-6	3 × 4-6	3 × 4-6			
Single-leg stride jump	114				3 × 4-6	3 × 4-6	3 × 4-6	3 × 4-6	3 × 4-6	3 × 4-6			
Stride jump crossover	115					3 × 4-6	3 × 4-6	3 × 4-6	3 × 4-6	3 × 4-6	3 × 4-6		
Power skipping	123				3 × 4-6	3 × 4-6	3 × 4-6	3 × 4-8	3 × 4-8				
Alternate-leg bound	131					2 × 4-6	3 × 4-6	3 × 4-6	3 × 6-8	3 × 8-10		3 × 8-12	
Incremental vertical hop	137						2 × 4-6	3 × 4-6	3 × 6-8		3 × 8-12		3 × 8-12
Side hop	138								2 × 4-6	3 × 6-8	3 × 6-8	3 × 6-10	3 × 6-10
Single-leg hop progression	143									2 × 4-6	3 × 4-6	3 × 4-6	3 × 4-6
Single-leg diagonal hop	145									2 × 3-6	3 × 3-6	3 × 3-6	3 × 3-6
Leg toss	91										2 × 3-6	4 × 3-6	4 × 3-6
Stepping two-arm overhead throw	72										2 × 3-6	4 × 3-6	4 × 3-6
Impact intensity			Low		Medium				High			Shock	

Table 9.2 Continuum Training for Baseball, Softball, and Cricket

		PROGRAM BASICS											
Exercise	Page #	Wk 1	Wk 2	Wk 3	Wk 4	Wk 5	Wk 6	Wk 7	Wk 8	Wk 9	Wk 10	Wk 11	Wk 12
Pogo	104	3 × 10	3 × 10	3 × 0	3 × 10								
Squat jump	105	2 × 4-6	3 × 4-6	3 × 6-8									
Medicine ball over and under, medicine ball half and full twist	88, 92, and 93	3 × 3	3 × 4	3 × 5	3 × 6	3 × 6							
Rocket jump and star jump	107 and 108	2 × 4-6	2 × 4-6	3 × 4-6		3 × 4-6							
Split jump and scissors jump	111 and 112	2 × 4-6		3 × 4-6	3 × 6-8	3 × 6-8	3 × 4-6						
Prancing	120	2 × 4-6	2 × 4-6	2 × 4-6	2 × 4-6	2 × 4-6							
Galloping	121	3 × 10	3 × 10	3 × 0	3 × 10	2 × 10	2 × 10	2 × 10	2 × 10	2 × 10	2 × 10	2 × 10	2 × 10
Fast skipping	122	3 × 10	3 × 10	3 × 10	3 × 10	2 × 10	2 × 10	2 × 10	2 × 10	2 × 10	2 × 10	2 × 10	2 × 10
Ankle flip	125	2 × 4-6	3 × 4-6	3 × 4-6	3 × 6-8	3 × 6-8	3 × 6-8	3 × 6-8	3 × 6-8	3 × 6-8	2 × 8-10	2 × 8-10	2 × 8-10
Single-leg stair bound	127		2 × 4-6	2 × 4-6	3 × 6-8		2 × 8-10	2 × 8-10		2 × 8-10			
Lateral bound (single response)	126			2 × 6-8	3 × 6-8	3 × 8-10	3 × 8-12			3 × 10-12			
Alternate-leg stair bound	130		2 × 6-8	3 × 6-8	3 × 8-10	3 × 8-12	3 × 8-12	3 × 8-12					
		DESIRABLES											
Bar twist	94	3 × 8-12	3 × 8-12	3 × 8-12	3 × 8-12	3 × 8-12	3 × 8-12						
Heavy bag stroke	76			3 × 8-12	3 × 8-12	3 × 8-12			3 × 8-12	3 × 8-12			
Sit-up throw	67			3 × 12-20	3 × 12-20		3 × 12-20	3 × 12-20		3 × 12-20			
Shovel toss progression	84				3 × 4-6	3 × 4-6	3 × 4-6	3 × 4-6	3 × 4-6	3 × 4-6			
Twist toss progression	95		3 × 6-12	3 × 6-12	3 × 6-12		3 × 6-12	3 × 6-12					
Horizontal swing	89		3 × 4-6	3 × 4-6	3 × 6-8	3 × 6-8		3 × 8-10	3 × 8-10				
Incline ricochet	148			2 × 6-10	2 × 6-10	2 × 6-10	3 × 6-12		3 × 6-12	3 × 6-12		3 × 6-12	
Knee-tuck jump	110			2 × 4-6		3 × 4-6	3 × 4-6	3 × 6-8	3 × 6-8		3 × 6-8		3 × 6-8
Double-leg slide kick	109			2 × 4-6	2 × 4-6	3 × 4-6	3 × 4-6	3 × 4-6		3 × 6-8	3 × 6-8	3 × 6-8	3 × 6-8
Power skipping	123			2 × 4-6	2 × 4-6		2 × 4-6	2 × 4-6		2 × 4-6	2 × 4-6	2 × 4-6	2 × 4-6
Double-leg hop progression	135						2-4 × 2	3-6 × 2	3-6 × 2	3-6 × 2		3-6 × 2	3-6 × 2
Side hop	138				2 × 3-6		2 × 3-6	2 × 3-6	2 × 3-6	3 × 3-6	3 × 3-6	3 × 3-6	3 × 3-6
Impact intensity			Low		Medium				High			Shock	

Table 9.3 Continuum Training for Baseball Pitchers

		PROGRAM BASICS											
Exercise	Page #	Wk 1	Wk 2	Wk 3	Wk 4	Wk 5	Wk 6	Wk 7	Wk 8	Wk 9	Wk 10	Wk 11	Wk 12
Pogo	104	3 × 10	3 × 10	3 × 10	3 × 10								
Squat jump	105	2 × 4-6	3 × 4-6	3 × 6-8									
Medicine ball over and under, medicine ball half and full twist	88, 92, and 93	3 × 3	3 × 4	3 × 5	3 × 6	3 × 6							
Rocket jump and star jump	107 and 108	2 × 4-6	2 × 4-6	3 × 4-6		3 × 4-6							
Split jump and scissors jump	111 and 112	2 × 4-6		3 × 4-6	3 × 6-8	3 × 6-8	3 × 4-6						
Prancing	120	2 × 4-6	2 × 4-6	2 × 4-6	2 × 4-6	2 × 4-6							
Galloping	121	3 × 10	3 × 10	3 × 10	3 × 10	2 × 10	2 × 10	2 × 10	2 × 10	2 × 10	2 × 10	2 × 10	2 × 10
Fast skipping	122	3 × 10	3 × 10	3 × 10	3 × 10	2 × 10	2 × 10	2 × 10	2 × 10	2 × 10	2 × 10	2 × 10	2 × 10
Ankle flip	125	2 × 4-6	3 × 4-6	3 × 4-6	3 × 6-8	3 × 6-8	3 × 6-8	3 × 6-8	3 × 6-8	3 × 6-8	2 × 8-10	2 × 8-10	2 × 8-10
Single-leg stair bound	127		2 × 4-6	2 × 4-6	3 × 6-8			2 × 8-10	2 × 8-10		2 × 8-10		
Lateral bound (single response)	126			2 × 6-8	3 × 6-8	3 × 8-10	3 × 8-12		3 × 10-12				
Alternate-leg stair bound	130		2 × 6-8	3 × 6-8	3 × 8-10	3 × 8-12	3 × 8-12	3 × 8-12					
		DESIRABLES											
Incline ricochet	148	3 × 8-12	3 × 8-12	3 × 8-12	3 × 8-12	3 × 8-12	3 × 8-12						
Bar twist	94	3 × 8-12	3 × 8-12	3 × 8-12	3 × 8-12	3 × 8-12		3 × 8-12					
Twist toss progression	95	3 × 12-20		3 × 12-20	3 × 12-20		3 × 12-20	3 × 12-20					
Heavy bag thrust	75		3 × 4-6	3 × 4-6	3 × 4-6	3 × 4-6	3 × 4-6	3 × 4-6					
Heavy bag stroke	76		3 × 6-12	3 × 6-12	3 × 6-12		3 × 6-12	3 × 6-12					
Shovel toss	84		3 × 4-6	3 × 4-6	3 × 6-8	3 × 6-8		3 × 8-10	3 × 8-10				
Scoop toss progression	85				3 × 4-6	3 × 4-6	3 × 4-6		3 × 6-8	3 × 6-8		3 × 6-8	
Shovel toss progression	84			2 × 4-6		3 × 4-6	3 × 4-6	3 × 6-8	3 × 6-8		3 × 6-8		3 × 6-8
Forward throw progression	68-73			2 × 4-6	2 × 4-6	3 × 4-6	3 × 4-6	3 × 4-6		3 × 6-8	3 × 6-8	3 × 6-8	3 × 6-8
Sit-up throw progression	67			2 × 10-20	2 × 10-20		2 × 10-20		2 × 10-20	2 × 10-20	2 × 10-20	2 × 10-20	2 × 10-20
Horizontal swing	89						2 × 8-12	2 × 8-12	2 × 8-12	2 × 8-12		2 × 8-12	2 × 8-12
Floor kip	99					2 × 3-6		2 × 3-6	2 × 3-6	3 × 3-6	3 × 3-6	3 × 3-6	3 × 3-6
Impact intensity			Low		Medium				High			Shock	

Table 9.4 Continuum Training for Volleyball

PROGRAM BASICS													
Exercise	Page #	Wk 1	Wk 2	Wk 3	Wk 4	Wk 5	Wk 6	Wk 7	Wk 8	Wk 9	Wk 10	Wk 11	Wk 12
Pogo	104	3 × 10	3 × 10	3 × 10	3 × 10								
Squat jump	105	2 × 4-6	3 × 4-6	3 × 6-8									
Medicine ball over and under, medicine ball half and full twist	88, 92, and 93	3 × 3	3 × 4	3 × 5	3 × 6	3 × 6							
Rocket jump and star jump	107 and 108	2 × 4-6	2 × 4-6	3 × 4-6		3 × 4-6							
Split jump and scissors jump	111 and 112	2 × 4-6		3 × 4-6	3 × 6-8	3 × 6-8	3 × 4-6						
Prancing	120	2 × 4-6	2 × 4-6	2 × 4-6	2 × 4-6	2 × 4-6							
Galloping	121	3 × 10	3 × 10	3 × 10	3 × 10	2 × 10	2 × 10	2 × 10	2 × 10	2 × 10	2 × 10	2 × 10	2 × 10
Fast skipping	122	3 × 10	3 × 10	3 × 10	3 × 10	2 × 10	2 × 10	2 × 10	2 × 10	2 × 10	2 × 10	2 × 10	2 × 10
Ankle flip	125	2 × 4-6	3 × 4-6	3 × 4-6	3 × 6-8	3 × 6-8	3 × 6-8	3 × 6-8	3 × 6-8	3 × 6-8	2 × 8-10	2 × 8-10	2 × 8-10
Single-leg stair bound	127		2 × 4-6	2 × 4-6	3 × 6-8			2 × 8-10	2 × 8-10		2 × 8-10		
Lateral bound (single response)	126		2 × 6-8	3 × 6-8	3 × 8-10	3 × 8-12	3 × 8-12		3 × 10-12				
Alternate-leg stair bound	130		2 × 6-8	3 × 6-8	3 × 8-10	3 × 8-12	3 × 8-12	3 × 8-12					
DESIRABLES													
Shovel toss	84	2 × 4-6	2 × 4-6	2 × 4-6	3 × 8-12		3 × 8-12						
Twist toss	95			3 × 8-12	3 × 8-12	3 × 8-12		3 × 8-12	3 × 8-12				
Sit-up throw	67			3 × 12-20	3 × 12-20	3 × 12-20	3 × 12-20	3 × 12-20	3 × 12-20	3 × 12-20			
Overhead throw progression	68-73				3 × 4-6	3 × 4-6	3 × 4-6	3 × 4-6	3 × 4-6	3 × 4-6			
Incline ricochet	148		3 × 4-6	3 × 4-6	3 × 4-6	3 × 6-12	3 × 6-12	3 × 6-12	3 × 6-12				
Lateral bound (single response)	126		3 × 4-6	3 × 4-6	3 × 4-6	3 × 4-6	3 × 4-8	3 × 4-8	3 × 4-8				
Power skipping	123			2 × 4-6	2 × 4-6	2 × 4-6	3 × 4-6	3 × 4-6	4 × 6-8	4 × 6-8		4 × 8-10	
Side hop	138					2 × 4-6	2 × 4-6	3 × 4-6	3 × 4-6		3 × 6-8		3 × 6-8
Incremental vertical hop	137					2 × 4-6	2 × 4-6	3 × 4-6		3 × 6-8	3 × 6-8	3 × 6-8	3 × 6-8
Side hop-sprint	139						2 × 4-6	2 × 4-6		2 × 4-6	2 × 4-6	2 × 4-6	2 × 4-6
Quick leap	116						2-4 × 2	3-6 × 2	3-6 × 2	3-6 × 2		3-6 × 2	3-6 × 2
Depth jump progression	117										2 × 3-6	3 × 3-6	3 × 3-6
Impact intensity			Low		Medium				High			Shock	

Table 9.5 Continuum Training for Cycling (Road, Criterium, Track)

		PROGRAM BASICS											
Exercise	Page #	Wk 1	Wk 2	Wk 3	Wk 4	Wk 5	Wk 6	Wk 7	Wk 8	Wk 9	Wk 10	Wk 11	Wk 12
Pogo	104	3 × 10	3 × 10	3 × 10	3 × 10								
Squat jump	105	2 × 4-6	3 × 4-6	3 × 6-8									
Medicine ball over and under, medicine ball half and full twist	88, 92, and 93	3 × 3	3 × 4	3 × 5	3 × 6	3 × 6							
Rocket jump and star jump	107 and 108	2 × 4-6	2 × 4-6	3 × 4-6		3 × 4-6							
Split jump and scissors jump	111 and 112	2 × 4-6		3 × 4-6	3 × 6-8	3 × 6-8	3 × 4-6						
Prancing	120	2 × 4-6	2 × 4-6	2 × 4-6	2 × 4-6	2 × 4-6							
Galloping	121	3 × 10	3 × 10	3 × 10	3 × 10	2 × 10	2 × 10	2 × 10	2 × 10	2 × 10	2 × 10	2 × 10	2 × 10
Fast skipping	122	3 × 10	3 × 10	3 × 10	3 × 10	2 × 10	2 × 10	2 × 10	2 × 10	2 × 10	2 × 10	2 × 10	2 × 10
Ankle flip	125	2 × 4-6	3 × 4-6	3 × 4-6	3 × 6-8	3 × 6-8	3 × 6-8	3 × 6-8	3 × 6-8	3 × 6-8	2 × 8-10	2 × 8-10	2 × 8-10
Single-leg stair bound	127		2 × 4-6	2 × 4-6	3 × 6-8		2 × 8-10	2 × 8-10		2 × 8-10			
Lateral bound (single response)	126			2 × 6-8	3 × 6-8	3 × 8-10	3 × 8-12		3 × 10-12				
Alternate-leg stair bound	130		2 × 6-8	3 × 6-8	3 × 8-10	3 × 8-12	3 × 8-12	3 × 8-12					
		DESIRABLES											
Incline ricochet	148		2 × 6-10	2 × 6-10	2 × 6-10		2 × 6-10	2 × 6-10	2 × 6-10				
Knee-tuck jump	110			3 × 4-6	3 × 4-6	3 × 4-6		3 × 4-6	3 × 4-6	3 × 4-6			
Single-leg stride jump	114				3 × 4-6	3 × 4-6	3 × 4-6		3 × 4-6	3 × 4-6	3 × 4-6		
Stride jump crossover	115							3 × 6-8	3 × 6-8	3 × 6-8	3 × 6-8	3 × 6-8	3 × 6-8
Double-leg hop progression	135					2 × 4-8	3 × 4-8	3 × 6-8		3 × 6-10	3 × 6-12	3 × 6-12	3 × 6-12
Alternate-leg bound	131					2 × 6-8	2 × 6-8		3 × 6-8		3 × 6-10	3 × 6-10	3 × 6-10
Single-leg hop progression	143							2 × 4-6	2 × 4-6	2 × 4-8		4 × 4-8	4 × 4-8
Depth jump	117										4-6 × 3	4-6 × 3	4-6 × 3
Impact intensity			Low		Medium				High			Shock	

165

Table 9.6 Continuum Training for Field Hockey

PROGRAM BASICS													
Exercise	Page #	Wk 1	Wk 2	Wk 3	Wk 4	Wk 5	Wk 6	Wk 7	Wk 8	Wk 9	Wk 10	Wk 11	Wk 12
Pogo	104	3 × 10	3 × 10	3 × 10	3 × 10								
Squat jump	105	2 × 4-6	3 × 4-6	3 × 6-8									
Medicine ball over and under, medicine ball half and full twist	88, 92, and 93	3 × 3	3 × 4	3 × 5	3 × 6	3 × 6							
Rocket jump and star jump	107 and 108	2 × 4-6	2 × 4-6	3 × 4-6		3 × 4-6							
Split jump and scissors jump	111 and 112	2 × 4-6		3 × 4-6	3 × 6-8	3 × 6-8	3 × 4-6						
Prancing	120	2 × 4-6	2 × 4-6	2 × 4-6	2 × 4-6	2 × 4-6							
Galloping	121	3 × 10	3 × 10	3 × 10	3 × 10	2 × 10	2 × 10	2 × 10	2 × 10	2 × 10	2 × 10	2 × 10	2 × 10
Fast skipping	122	3 × 10	3 × 10	3 × 10	3 × 10	2 × 10	2 × 10	2 × 10	2 × 10	2 × 10	2 × 10	2 × 10	2 × 10
Ankle flip	125	2 × 4-6	3 × 4-6	3 × 4-6	3 × 6-8	3 × 6-8	3 × 6-8	3 × 6-8	3 × 6-8	3 × 6-8	2 × 8-10	2 × 8-10	2 × 8-10
Single-leg stair bound	127		2 × 4-6	2 × 4-6	3 × 6-8		2 × 8-10	2 × 8-10		2 × 8-10			
Lateral bound (single response)	126			2 × 6-8	3 × 6-8	3 × 8-10	3 × 8-12		3 × 10-12				
Alternate-leg stair bound	130		2 × 6-8	3 × 6-8	3 × 8-10	3 × 8-12	3 × 8-12	3 × 8-12					
DESIRABLES													
Incline ricochet	148			3 × 8-12	3 × 8-12	3 × 8-12		3 × 8-12	3 × 8-12				
Knee-tuck jump	110			3 × 4-6	3 × 4-6	3 × 4-6	3 × 4-6	3 × 4-6	3 × 4-6	3 × 4-6			
Single-leg stride jump	114				3 × 4-6	3 × 4-6	3 × 4-6	3 × 4-6	3 × 4-6	3 × 4-6			
Stride jump crossover	115					3 × 4-6	3 × 4-6	3 × 4-6	3 × 4-6	3 × 4-6	3 × 4-6		
Power skipping	123				3 × 4-6	3 × 4-6	3 × 4-6	3 × 4-8	3 × 4-8				
Alternate-leg bound	131					2 × 4-6	3 × 4-6	3 × 4-6	3 × 6-8	3 × 8-10		3 × 8-12	
Incremental vertical hop	137						2 × 4-6	3 × 4-6	3 × 6-8		3 × 8-12		3 × 8-12
Side hop	138								2 × 4-6	3 × 6-8	3 × 6-8	3 × 6-10	3 × 6-10
Single-leg hop progression	143									2 × 4-6	3 × 4-6	3 × 4-6	3 × 4-6
Single-leg diagonal hop	145									2 × 3-6	3 × 3-6	3 × 3-6	3 × 3-6
Leg toss	91										2 × 3-6	4 × 3-6	4 × 3-6
Stepping two-arm overhead throw	72										2 × 3-6	4 × 3-6	4 × 3-6
Impact intensity			Low		Medium				High			Shock	

Table 9.7 Continuum Training for Basketball and Netball

Exercise	Page #	Wk 1	Wk 2	Wk 3	Wk 4	Wk 5	Wk 6	Wk 7	Wk 8	Wk 9	Wk 10	Wk 11	Wk 12
PROGRAM BASICS													
Pogo	104	3 × 10	3 × 10	3 × 10	3 × 10								
Squat jump	105	2 × 4-6	3 × 4-6	3 × 6-8									
Medicine ball over and under, medicine ball half and full twist	88, 92, and 93	3 × 3	3 × 4	3 × 5	3 × 6	3 × 6							
Rocket jump and star jump	107 and 108	2 × 4-6	2 × 4-6	3 × 4-6		3 × 4-6							
Split jump and scissors jump	111 and 112	2 × 4-6		3 × 4-6	3 × 6-8	3 × 6-8	3 × 4-6						
Prancing	120	2 × 4-6	2 × 4-6	2 × 4-6	2 × 4-6	2 × 4-6							
Galloping	121	3 × 10	3 × 10	3 × 10	3 × 10	2 × 10	2 × 10	2 × 10	2 × 10	2 × 10	2 × 10	2 × 10	2 × 10
Fast skipping	122	3 × 10	3 × 10	3 × 10	3 × 10	2 × 10	2 × 10	2 × 10	2 × 10	2 × 10	2 × 10	2 × 10	2 × 10
Ankle flip	125	2 × 4-6	3 × 4-6	3 × 4-6	3 × 6-8	3 × 6-8	3 × 6-8	3 × 6-8	3 × 6-8	3 × 6-8	2 × 8-10	2 × 8-10	2 × 8-10
Single-leg stair bound	127		2 × 4-6	2 × 4-6	3 × 6-8		2 × 8-10	2 × 8-10		2 × 8-10			
Lateral bound (single response)	126			2 × 6-8	3 × 6-8	3 × 8-10	3 × 8-12		3 × 10-12				
Alternate-leg stair bound	130		2 × 6-8	3 × 6-8	3 × 8-10	3 × 8-12	3 × 8-12	3 × 8-12					
DESIRABLES													
Scoop toss progression	85	2 × 4-6	2 × 4-6	2 × 4-6	3 × 8-12		3 × 8-12						
Medicine ball full twist	93			3 × 8-12	3 × 8-12	3 × 8-12		3 × 8-12	3 × 8-12				
Medicine ball chest pass	65			3 × 4-6	3 × 4-6	3 × 4-6	3 × 4-6	3 × 4-6	3 × 4-6	3 × 4-6			
Supine two-arm overhead throw	69				3 × 4-6	3 × 4-6	3 × 4-6	3 × 4-6	3 × 4-6	3 × 4-6			
Lateral bound	126					3 × 4-6	3 × 4-6	3 × 4-6	3 × 4-6	3 × 4-6	3 × 4-6		
Incline ricochet	148				3 × 4-6	3 × 4-6	3 × 4-6	3 × 4-8	3 × 4-8				
Double-leg hop progression	135					2 × 4-6	3 × 4-6	3 × 4-6	4 × 6-8	4 × 6-8		4 × 8-10	
Side hop	138						2 × 4-6	3 × 4-6	3 × 4-6		3 × 6-8		3 × 6-8
Incremental vertical hop	137							2 × 4-6	4 × 4-6	4 × 4-6	6 × 4-6	6 × 4-6	
Side hop-sprint	139									2-4 × 4-8	2-4 × 4-8	2-4 × 4-8	2-4 × 4-8
Double-leg hop	135									2-4 × 3-6	2-4 × 3-6	2-4 × 3-6	2-4 × 3-6
Depth jump progression	117									2 × 3-6	3 × 3-6	3 × 3-6	
Impact intensity			Low		Medium				High			Shock	

Table 9.8 Continuum Training for Crew Rowing

PROGRAM BASICS													
Exercise	Page #	Wk 1	Wk 2	Wk 3	Wk 4	Wk 5	Wk 6	Wk 7	Wk 8	Wk 9	Wk 10	Wk 11	Wk 12
Pogo	104	3 × 10	3 × 10	3 × 10	3 × 10								
Squat jump	105	2 × 4-6	3 × 4-6	3 × 6-8									
Medicine ball chest pass (kneeling)	65	2 × 4-6	3 × 4-6	3 × 6	3 × 6								2 × 3-5
Rocket jump and star jump	107 and 108	2 × 4-6	2 × 4-6	3 × 4-6		3 × 4-6							
Shovel toss	84	2 × 4-6		3 × 4-6	3 × 6	3 × 6	3 × 6						
Prancing	120	2 × 4-6	2 × 4-6	2 × 4-6	2 × 4-6	2 × 4-6							
Galloping	121	3 × 10	3 × 10	3 × 10	3 × 10	2 × 10	2 × 10	2 × 10	2 × 10	2 × 10	2 × 10	2 × 10	2 × 10
Fast skipping	122	3 × 10	3 × 10	3 × 10	3 × 10	2 × 10	2 × 10	2 × 10	2 × 10	2 × 10	2 × 10	2 × 10	2 × 10
Ankle flip	125	2 × 4-6	3 × 4-6	3 × 4-6	3 × 6-8	3 × 6-8	3 × 6-8	3 × 6-8	3 × 6-8	3 × 6-8	2 × 8-10	2 × 8-10	2 × 8-10
Double-leg incline bound	128		2 × 4-6	2 × 4-6	3 × 6-8		3 × 6-8	3 × 6-8		3 × 6-8			
Lateral bound (single response)	126			2 × 6-8	3 × 6-8	3 × 8-10	3 × 8-12		3 × 10-12				
Alternate-leg stair bound	130		2 × 6-8	3 × 6-8	3 × 8-10	3 × 8-12	3 × 8-12	3 × 8-12					
DESIRABLES													
Scoop toss	85	3 × 3-6	3 × 3-6		3 × 3-6	3 × 3-6	3 × 3-6						3 × 3-6
Shovel toss	84			3 × 3-6	3 × 3-6	3 × 3-6		3 × 3-6	3 × 3-6	3 × 3-6			
Knee-tuck jump	110			3 × 3-6	3 × 3-6	3 × 3-6		3 × 3-6	3 × 3-6	3 × 3-6			
Incremental vertical hop	137				3 × 3-6	3 × 3-6	3 × 3-6		3 × 3-6	3 × 3-6	3 × 3-6		
Bar kip-up	98				2 × 3-6	2 × 3-6	2 × 3-6		3 × 3-6	3 × 3-6	3 × 3-6		
Vertical swing	90				2 × 4-6	2 × 4-6	3 × 6-8		3 × 6-8	3 × 6-8		3 × 6-8	
Floor kip	99					3 × 1	3 × 1	3 × 1	3 × 1		3 × 1	3 × 1	3 × 1
Quick leap	116				4-8 × 1-2	4-8 × 1-2	4-8 × 1-2	4-8 × 1-2		4-8 × 1-2	4-8 × 1-2	4-8 × 1-2	4-8 × 1-2
Multiple hops to overhead throw	83						2 × 3-6	2 × 3-6	3 × 3-6		3 × 3-6	3 × 6	3 × 6
Double-leg speed hop	136						2 × 3-6	2 × 3-6	3 × 3-6		3 × 3-6	3 × 6	3 × 6
Depth jump	117									4-8 × 3-6	4-8 × 3-6	4-8 × 3-6	4-8 × 3-6
Depth jump leap	119										3-6 × 3-5	3-6 × 3-5	3-6 × 3-5
Impact intensity			Low		Medium				High			Shock	

Table 9.9 Continuum Training for American Football Linemen

PROGRAM BASICS													
Exercise	Page #	Wk 1	Wk 2	Wk 3	Wk 4	Wk 5	Wk 6	Wk 7	Wk 8	Wk 9	Wk 10	Wk 11	Wk 12
Pogo	104	3 × 10	3 × 10	3 × 10	3 × 10								
Squat jump	105	2 × 4-6	3 × 4-6	3 × 6-8									
Medicine ball over and under, medicine ball half and full twist	88, 92, and 93	3 × 3	3 × 4	3 × 5	3 × 6	3 × 6							
Rocket jump and star jump	107 and 108	2 × 4-6	2 × 4-6	3 × 4-6		3 × 4-6							
Split jump and scissors jump	111 and 112	2 × 4-6		3 × 4-6	3 × 6-8	3 × 6-8	3 × 4-6						
Prancing	120	2 × 4-6	2 × 4-6	2 × 4-6	2 × 4-6	2 × 4-6							
Galloping	121	3 × 10	3 × 10	3 × 10	3 × 10	2 × 10	2 × 10	2 × 10	2 × 10	2 × 10	2 × 10	2 × 10	2 × 10
Fast skipping	122	3 × 10	3 × 10	3 × 10	3 × 10	2 × 10	2 × 10	2 × 10	2 × 10	2 × 10	2 × 10	2 × 10	2 × 10
Ankle flip	125	2 × 4-6	3 × 4-6	3 × 4-6	3 × 6-8	3 × 6-8	3 × 6-8	3 × 6-8	3 × 6-8	3 × 6-8	2 × 8-10	2 × 8-10	2 × 8-10
Single-leg stair bound	127		2 × 4-6	2 × 4-6	3 × 6-8		2 × 8-10	2 × 8-10		2 × 8-10			
Lateral bound (single response)	126			2 × 6-8	3 × 6-8	3 × 8-10	3 × 8-12		3 × 10-12				
Alternate-leg stair bound	130		2 × 6-8	3 × 6-8	3 × 8-10	3 × 8-12	3 × 8-12	3 × 8-12					
DESIRABLES													
Leap progression	118 and 119			3 × 4-6	3 × 4-6	3 × 6-8	3 × 6-8	3 × 6-8					
Incline ricochet	148			3 × 8-12	3 × 8-12	3 × 8-12		3 × 8-12	3 × 8-12	3 × 8-12			
Medicine ball chest pass progression	65				3 × 4-6	3 × 4-6	3 × 4-6	3 × 4-6	3 × 4-6	3 × 4-6			
Shovel toss progression	84					3 × 4-6	3 × 4-6	3 × 4-6	3 × 4-6	3 × 4-6	3 × 4-6		
Knee-tuck jump	110				3 × 4-6	3 × 4-6	3 × 4-6	3 × 4-8	3 × 4-8	3 × 4-8			
Power skipping	123					2 × 4-6	3 × 4-6	3 × 4-6	4 × 6-8		4 × 6-8		4 × 8-10
Double-leg hop progression	135					2 × 4-6	2 × 4-6	3 × 4-6	3 × 4-6	3 × 6-8	3 × 6-8	3 × 6-8	3 × 6-8
Side hop-sprint	139								2 × 4-6	4 × 4-6	4 × 4-6	6 × 4-6	6 × 4-6
Side hop	138								3 × 4-6	3 × 6-8	3 × 6-8	3 × 6-8	3 × 6-8
Alternate-leg bound	131								3 × 4-6	3 × 6-8		3 × 6-8	
Depth jump progression	117									3 × 3	3 × 3	3 × 3	
Depth leap progression	118										3 × 3	3 × 3	3 × 3
Impact intensity			Low			Medium				High			Shock	

169

Table 9.10 Continuum Training for American Football Backs

PROGRAM BASICS													
Exercise	Page #	Wk 1	Wk 2	Wk 3	Wk 4	Wk 5	Wk 6	Wk 7	Wk 8	Wk 9	Wk 10	Wk 11	Wk 12
Pogo	104	3 × 10	3 × 10	3 × 10	3 × 10								
Squat jump	105	2 × 4-6	3 × 4-6	3 × 6-8									
Medicine ball over and under, medicine ball half and full twist	88, 92, and 93	3 × 3	3 × 4	3 × 5	3 × 6	3 × 6							
Rocket jump and star jump	107 and 108	2 × 4-6	2 × 4-6	3 × 4-6		3 × 4-6							
Split jump and scissors jump	111 and 112	2 × 4-6		3 × 4-6	3 × 6-8	3 × 6-8	3 × 4-6						
Prancing	120	2 × 4-6	2 × 4-6	2 × 4-6	2 × 4-6	2 × 4-6							
Galloping	121	3 × 10	3 × 10	3 × 10	3 × 10	2 × 10	2 × 10	2 × 10	2 × 10	2 × 10	2 × 10	2 × 10	2 × 10
Fast skipping	122	3 × 10	3 × 10	3 × 10	3 × 10	2 × 10	2 × 10	2 × 10	2 × 10	2 × 10	2 × 10	2 × 10	2 × 10
Ankle flip	125	2 × 4-6	3 × 4-6	3 × 4-6	3 × 6-8	3 × 6-8	3 × 6-8	3 × 6-8	3 × 6-8	3 × 6-8	2 × 8-10	2 × 8-10	2 × 8-10
Single-leg stair bound	127		2 × 4-6	2 × 4-6	3 × 6-8		2 × 8-10	2 × 8-10		2 × 8-10			
Lateral bound (single response)	126			2 × 6-8	3 × 6-8	3 × 8-10	3 × 8-12		3 × 10-12				
Alternate-leg stair bound	130		2 × 6-8	3 × 6-8	3 × 8-10	3 × 8-12	3 × 8-12	3 × 8-12					
DESIRABLES													
Incline ricochet	148			3 × 8-12	3 × 8-12	3 × 8-12		3 × 8-12	3 × 8-12				
Knee-tuck jump	110			3 × 4-6	3 × 4-6	3 × 4-6	3 × 4-6	3 × 4-6	3 × 4-6	3 × 4-6			
Double-leg slide kick	109				3 × 4-6	3 × 4-6	3 × 4-6	3 × 4-6	3 × 4-6	3 × 4-6			
Double-leg hop progression	135					3 × 4-6	3 × 4-6	3 × 4-6	3 × 4-6	3 × 4-6	3 × 4-6		
Side hop	138				3 × 4-6	3 × 4-6	3 × 4-6	3 × 4-8	3 × 4-8				
Power skipping	123					2 × 4-6	3 × 4-6	3 × 4-6	4 × 6-8	4 × 6-8		4 × 8-10	
Alternate-leg bound	131						2 × 4-6	3 × 4-6	3 × 4-6		3 × 6-8		3 × 6-8
Extended skipping	124								2 × 4-6	4 × 4-6	4 × 4-6	6 × 4-6	6 × 4-6
Depth jump	117									2-4 × 4-8	2-4 × 4-8	2-4 × 4-8	2-4 × 4-8
Depth leap	118									2-4 × 3-6	2-4 × 3-6	2-4 × 3-6	2-4 × 3-6
Single-leg hop progression	143										2 × 3-6	3 × 3-6	3 × 3-6
Single-leg lateral hop progression	146										2 × 3-6	3 × 3-6	3 × 3-6
Impact intensity			Low		Medium				High			Shock	

Table 9.11 Continuum Training for American Football Quarterbacks

Exercise	Page #	Wk 1	Wk 2	Wk 3	Wk 4	Wk 5	Wk 6	Wk 7	Wk 8	Wk 9	Wk 10	Wk 11	Wk 12
PROGRAM BASICS													
Pogo	104	3 × 10	3 × 10	3 × 10	3 × 10								
Squat jump	105	2 × 4-6	3 × 4-6	3 × 6-8									
Medicine ball over and under, medicine ball half and full twist	88, 92, and 93	3 × 3	3 × 4	3 × 5	3 × 6	3 × 6							
Rocket jump and star jump	107 and 108	2 × 4-6	2 × 4-6	3 × 4-6		3 × 4-6							
Split jump and scissors jump	111 and 112	2 × 4-6		3 × 4-6	3 × 6-8	3 × 6-8	3 × 4-6						
Prancing	120	2 × 4-6	2 × 4-6	2 × 4-6	2 × 4-6	2 × 4-6							
Galloping	121	3 × 10	3 × 10	3 × 10	3 × 10	2 × 10	2 × 10	2 × 10	2 × 10	2 × 10	2 × 10	2 × 10	2 × 10
Fast skipping	122	3 × 10	3 × 10	3 × 10	3 × 10	2 × 10	2 × 10	2 × 10	2 × 10	2 × 10	2 × 10	2 × 10	2 × 10
Ankle flip	125	2 × 4-6	3 × 4-6	3 × 4-6	3 × 6-8	3 × 6-8	3 × 6-8	3 × 6-8	3 × 6-8	3 × 6-8	2 × 8-10	2 × 8-10	2 × 8-10
Single-leg stair bound	127		2 × 4-6	2 × 4-6	3 × 6-8		2 × 8-10	2 × 8-10			2 × 8-10		
Lateral bound (single response)	126			2 × 6-8	3 × 6-8	3 × 8-10	3 × 8-12		3 × 10-12				
Alternate-leg stair bound	130		2 × 6-8	3 × 6-8	3 × 8-10	3 × 8-12	3 × 8-12	3 × 8-12					
DESIRABLES													
Incline ricochet	148	3 × 8-12	3 × 8-12	3 × 8-12	3 × 8-12	3 × 8-12	3 × 8-12						
Bar twist	94	3 × 8-12	3 × 8-12	3 × 8-12	3 × 8-12	3 × 8-12		3 × 8-12					
Twist toss progression	95	3 × 12-20		3 × 12-20	3 × 12-20		3 × 12-20	3 × 12-20					
Heavy bag thrust	75		3 × 4-6	3 × 4-6	3 × 4-6	3 × 4-6	3 × 4-6	3 × 4-6					
Heavy bag stroke	76		3 × 6-12	3 × 6-12	3 × 6-12		3 × 6-12	3 × 6-12					
Shovel toss	84		3 × 4-6	3 × 4-6	3 × 6-8	3 × 6-8		3 × 8-10	3 × 8-10				
Scoop toss progression	85				3 × 4-6	3 × 4-6	3 × 4-6		3 × 6-8	3 × 6-8		3 × 6-8	
Shovel toss progression	84			2 × 4-6		3 × 4-6	3 × 4-6	3 × 6-8	3 × 6-8		3 × 6-8		3 × 6-8
Forward throw progression	68-73			2 × 4-6	2 × 4-6	3 × 4-6	3 × 4-6	3 × 4-6		3 × 6-8	3 × 6-8	3 × 6-8	3 × 6-8
Sit-up throw progression	67	2 × 10-20	2 × 10-20		2 × 10-20		2 × 10-20		2 × 10-20	2 × 10-20	2 × 10-20	2 × 10-20	2 × 10-20
Horizontal swing	89						2 × 8-12	2 × 8-12	2 × 8-12	2 × 8-12		2 × 8-12	2 × 8-12
Floor kip	99					2 × 3-6		2 × 3-6	2 × 3-6	3 × 3-6	3 × 3-6	3 × 3-6	3 × 3-6
Impact intensity			Low		Medium				High			Shock	

Table 9.12 Continuum Training for American Football Punters and Kickers

PROGRAM BASICS													
Exercise	Page #	Wk 1	Wk 2	Wk 3	Wk 4	Wk 5	Wk 6	Wk 7	Wk 8	Wk 9	Wk 10	Wk 11	Wk 12
Pogo	104	3 × 10	3 × 10	3 × 10	3 × 10								
Squat jump	105	2 × 4-6	3 × 4-6	3 × 6-8									
Medicine ball over and under, medicine ball half and full twist	88, 92, and 93	3 × 3	3 × 4	3 × 5	3 × 6	3 × 6							
Rocket jump and star jump	107 and 108	2 × 4-6	2 × 4-6	3 × 4-6		3 × 4-6							
Split jump and scissors jump	111 and 112	2 × 4-6		3 × 4-6	3 × 6-8	3 × 6-8	3 × 4-6						
Prancing	120	2 × 4-6	2 × 4-6	2 × 4-6	2 × 4-6	2 × 4-6							
Galloping	121	3 × 10	3 × 10	3 × 10	3 × 10	2 × 10	2 × 10	2 × 10	2 × 10	2 × 10	2 × 10	2 × 10	2 × 10
Fast skipping	122	3 × 10	3 × 10	3 × 10	3 × 10	2 × 10	2 × 10	2 × 10	2 × 10	2 × 10	2 × 10	2 × 10	2 × 10
Ankle flip	125	2 × 4-6	3 × 4-6	3 × 4-6	3 × 6-8	3 × 6-8	3 × 6-8	3 × 6-8	3 × 6-8	3 × 6-8	2 × 8-10	2 × 8-10	2 × 8-10
Single-leg stair bound	127		2 × 4-6	2 × 4-6	3 × 6-8		2 × 8-10	2 × 8-10		2 × 8-10			
Lateral bound (single response)	126			2 × 6-8	3 × 6-8	3 × 8-10	3 × 8-12		3 × 10-12				
Alternate-leg stair bound	130		2 × 6-8	3 × 6-8	3 × 8-10	3 × 8-12	3 × 8-12	3 × 8-12					
DESIRABLES													
Incline ricochet	148			3 × 8-12	3 × 8-12	3 × 8-12		3 × 8-12	3 × 8-12				
Knee-tuck jump	110			3 × 4-6	3 × 4-6	3 × 4-6	3 × 4-6	3 × 4-6	3 × 4-6	3 × 4-6			
Single-leg stride jump	114				3 × 4-6	3 × 4-6	3 × 4-6	3 × 4-6	3 × 4-6	3 × 4-6			
Stride jump crossover	115					3 × 4-6	3 × 4-6	3 × 4-6	3 × 4-6	3 × 4-6	3 × 4-6		
Power skipping	123				3 × 4-6	3 × 4-6	3 × 4-6	3 × 4-8	3 × 4-8				
Alternate-leg bound	131					2 × 4-6	3 × 4-6	3 × 4-6	3 × 6-8	3 × 8-10		3 × 8-12	
Incremental vertical hop	137						2 × 4-6	3 × 4-6	3 × 6-8		3 × 8-12		3 × 8-12
Side hop	138								2 × 4-6	3 × 6-8	3 × 6-8	3 × 6-10	3 × 6-10
Single-leg hop progression	143									2 × 4-6	3 × 4-6	3 × 4-6	3 × 4-6
Single-leg diagonal hop	145									2 × 3-6	3 × 3-6	3 × 3-6	3 × 3-6
Leg toss	91										2 × 3-6	4 × 3-6	4 × 3-6
Stepping two-arm overhead throw	72										2 × 3-6	4 × 3-6	4 × 3-6
Impact intensity			Low		Medium				High			Shock	

Table 9.13 Continuum Training for Alpine Skiing

		PROGRAM BASICS											
Exercise	Page #	Wk 1	Wk 2	Wk 3	Wk 4	Wk 5	Wk 6	Wk 7	Wk 8	Wk 9	Wk 10	Wk 11	Wk 12
Pogo	104	3 × 10	3 × 10	3 × 10	3 × 10								
Squat jump	105	2 × 4-6	3 × 4-6	3 × 6-8									
Medicine ball over and under, medicine ball half and full twist	88, 92, and 93	3 × 3	3 × 4	3 × 5	3 × 6	3 × 6							
Rocket jump and star jump	107 and 108	2 × 4-6	2 × 4-6	3 × 4-6		3 × 4-6							
Split jump and scissors jump	111 and 112	2 × 4-6		3 × 4-6	3 × 6-8	3 × 6-8	3 × 4-6						
Prancing	120	2 × 4-6	2 × 4-6	2 × 4-6	2 × 4-6	2 × 4-6							
Galloping	121	3 × 10	3 × 10	3 × 10	3 × 10	2 × 10	2 × 10	2 × 10	2 × 10	2 × 10	2 × 10	2 × 10	2 × 10
Fast skipping	122	3 × 10	3 × 10	3 × 10	3 × 10	2 × 10	2 × 10	2 × 10	2 × 10	2 × 10	2 × 10	2 × 10	2 × 10
Ankle flip	125	2 × 4-6	3 × 4-6	3 × 4-6	3 × 6-8	3 × 6-8	3 × 6-8	3 × 6-8	3 × 6-8	3 × 6-8	2 × 8-10	2 × 8-10	2 × 8-10
Single-leg stair bound	127		2 × 4-6	2 × 4-6	3 × 6-8		2 × 8-10	2 × 8-10		2 × 8-10			
Lateral bound (single response)	126			2 × 6-8	3 × 6-8	3 × 8-10	3 × 8-12		3 × 10-12				
Alternate-leg stair bound	130		2 × 6-8	3 × 6-8	3 × 8-10	3 × 8-12	3 × 8-12	3 × 8-12					
		DESIRABLES											
Incline ricochet	148			3 × 8-12	3 × 8-12	3 × 8-12		3 × 8-12	3 × 8-12				
Knee-tuck jump	110			3 × 4-6	3 × 4-6	3 × 4-6	3 × 4-6	3 × 4-6	3 × 4-6	3 × 4-6			
Single-leg stride jump	114				3 × 4-6	3 × 4-6	3 × 4-6	3 × 4-6	3 × 4-6	3 × 4-6			
Stride jump crossover	115					3 × 4-6	3 × 4-6	3 × 4-6	3 × 4-6	3 × 4-6	3 × 4-6		
Quick leap	116				3 × 4-6	3 × 4-6	3 × 4-6	3 × 4-8	3 × 4-8				
Double-leg incline bound	128					2 × 4-6	3 × 4-6	3 × 4-6	4 × 6-8	4 × 6-8		4 × 8-10	
Alternate-leg bound	131						2 × 4-6	3 × 4-6	3 × 6-8		3 × 8-12		3 × 8-12
Double-leg hop progression	135								2 × 4-6	3 × 6-8	3 × 6-8	3 × 6-10	3 × 6-10
Side hop	138									2 × 4-6	3 × 4-6	3 × 4-6	3 × 4-6
Incremental vertical hop	137									2 × 3-6	3 × 3-6	3 × 3-6	3 × 3-6
Single-leg hop progression	143										2 × 3-6	4 × 3-6	4 × 3-6
Single-leg diagonal hop	145										2 × 3-6	4 × 3-6	4 × 3-6
Impact intensity			Low		Medium				High			Shock	

Table 9.14 Continuum Training for Nordic Skiing

Exercise	Page #	Wk 1	Wk 2	Wk 3	Wk 4	Wk 5	Wk 6	Wk 7	Wk 8	Wk 9	Wk 10	Wk 11	Wk 12
PROGRAM BASICS													
Pogo	104	3 × 10	3 × 10	3 × 10	3 × 10								
Squat jump	105	2 × 4-6	3 × 4-6	3 × 6-8									
Medicine ball over and under, medicine ball half and full twist	88, 92, and 93	3 × 3	3 × 4	3 × 5	3 × 6	3 × 6							
Rocket jump and star jump	107 and 108	2 × 4-6	2 × 4-6	3 × 4-6		3 × 4-6							
Split jump and scissors jump	111 and 112	2 × 4-6		3 × 4-6	3 × 6-8	3 × 6-8	3 × 4-6						
Prancing	120	2 × 4-6	2 × 4-6	2 × 4-6	2 × 4-6	2 × 4-6							
Galloping	121	3 × 10	3 × 10	3 × 10	3 × 10	2 × 10	2 × 10	2 × 10	2 × 10	2 × 10	2 × 10	2 × 10	2 × 10
Fast skipping	122	3 × 10	3 × 10	3 × 10	3 × 10	2 × 10	2 × 10	2 × 10	2 × 10	2 × 10	2 × 10	2 × 10	2 × 10
Ankle flip	125	2 × 4-6	3 × 4-6	3 × 4-6	3 × 6-8	3 × 6-8	3 × 6-8	3 × 6-8	3 × 6-8	3 × 6-8	2 × 8-10	2 × 8-10	2 × 8-10
Single-leg stair bound	127		2 × 4-6	2 × 4-6	3 × 6-8		2 × 8-10	2 × 8-10		2 × 8-10			
Lateral bound (single response)	126			2 × 6-8	3 × 6-8	3 × 8-10	3 × 8-12		3 × 10-12				
Alternate-leg stair bound	130		2 × 6-8	3 × 6-8	3 × 8-10	3 × 8-12	3 × 8-12	3 × 8-12					
DESIRABLES													
Sit-up throw progression	67	2 × 3-6	3 × 3-6	3 × 5-8	3 × 6-12	3 × 6-12	3 × 6-12						
Vertical swing	90		3 × 6-12	3 × 6-12	3 × 6-12	3 × 6-12	3 × 6-12	3 × 6-12					
Arm swing	74			3 × 6-12	3 × 6-12	3 × 6-12	3 × 6-12	3 × 6-12	3 × 6-12	3 × 6-12			
Incline ricochet	148			3 × 8-12	3 × 8-12	3 × 8-12		3 × 8-12	3 × 8-12				
Knee-tuck jump	110			3 × 4-6	3 × 4-6	3 × 4-6	3 × 4-6	3 × 4-6	3 × 4-6	3 × 4-6			
Single-leg stride jump	114				3 × 4-6	3 × 4-6	3 × 4-6	3 × 4-6	3 × 4-6	3 × 4-6			
Stride jump crossover	115					3 × 4-6	3 × 4-6	3 × 4-6	3 × 4-6	3 × 4-6	3 × 4-6		
Quick leap	116				3 × 4-6	3 × 4-6	3 × 4-6	3 × 4-8	3 × 4-8				
Double-leg incline bound	128					2 × 4-6	3 × 4-6	3 × 4-6	4 × 6-8	4 × 6-8		4 × 10	
Alternate-leg bound	131						2 × 4-6	3 × 4-6	3 × 6-8		3 × 8-12		3 × 8-12
Single-leg hop progression	143										2 × 3-6	4 × 6	4 × 6
Single-leg diagonal hop	145										2 × 3-6	4 × 3-6	4 × 3-6
Impact intensity			Low		Medium				High			Shock	

174

Table 9.15 Continuum Training for Lacrosse

PROGRAM BASICS													
Exercise	Page #	Wk 1	Wk 2	Wk 3	Wk 4	Wk 5	Wk 6	Wk 7	Wk 8	Wk 9	Wk 10	Wk 11	Wk 12
Pogo	104	3×10	3×0	3×10	3×10								
Squat jump	105	2×4-6	3×4-6	3×6-8									
Medicine ball over and under, medicine ball half and full twist	88, 92, and 93	3×3	3×4	3×5	3×6	3×6							
Rocket jump and star jump	107 and 108	2×4-6	2×4-6	3×4-6		3×4-6							
Split jump and scissors jump	111 and 112	2×4-6		3×4-6	3×6-8	3×6-8	3×4-6						
Prancing	120	2×4-6	2×4-6	2×4-6	2×4-6	2×4-6							
Galloping	121	3×10	3×10	3×10	3×10	2×10	2×10	2×10	2×10	2×10	2×10	2×10	2×10
Fast skipping	122	3×10	3×10	3×10	3×10	2×10	2×10	2×10	2×10	2×10	2×10	2×10	2×10
Ankle flip	125	2×4-6	3×4-6	3×4-6	3×6-8	3×6-8	3×6-8	3×6-8	3×6-8	3×6-8	2×8-10	2×8-10	2×8-10
Single-leg stair bound	127		2×4-6	2×4-6	3×6-8			2×8-10	2×8-10		2×8-10		
Lateral bound (single response)	126			2×6-8	3×6-8	3×8-10	3×8-12		3×10-12				
Alternate-leg stair bound	130		2×6-8	3×6-8	3×8-10	3×8-12	3×8-12	3×8-12					
DESIRABLES													
Incline ricochet	148			3×8-12	3×8-12	3×8-12		3×8-12	3×8-12				
Knee-tuck jump	110			3×4-6	3×4-6	3×4-6	3×4-6	3×4-6	3×4-6	3×4-6			
Single-leg stride jump	114				3×4-6	3×4-6	3×4-6	3×4-6	3×4-6	3×4-6			
Stride jump crossover	115					3×4-6	3×4-6	3×4-6	3×4-6	3×4-6	3×4-6		
Power skipping	123				3×4-6	3×4-6	3×4-6	3×4-8	3×4-8				
Alternate-leg bound	131					2×4-6	3×4-6	3×4-6	3×6-8	3×8-10		3×8-12	
Incremental vertical hop	137						2×4-6	3×4-6	3×6-8		3×8-12		3×8-12
Side hop	138								2×4-6	3×6-8	3×6-8	3×6-10	3×6-10
Single-leg hop progression	143									2×4-6	3×4-6	3×4-6	3×4-6
Single-leg diagonal hop	145									2×3-6	3×3-6	3×3-6	3×3-6
Leg toss	91										2×3-6	4×3-6	4×3-6
Stepping two-arm overhead throw	72										2×3-6	4×3-6	4×3-6
Impact intensity			Low		Medium				High			Shock	

175

Table 9.16 Continuum Training for Tennis, Racquetball, Squash, and Handball

Exercise	Page #	Wk 1	Wk 2	Wk 3	Wk 4	Wk 5	Wk 6	Wk 7	Wk 8	Wk 9	Wk 10	Wk 11	Wk 12
PROGRAM BASICS													
Pogo	104	3×10	3×10	3×10	3×10								
Squat jump	105	2×4-6	3×4-6	3×6-8									
Medicine ball over and under, medicine ball half and full twist	88, 92, and 93	3×3	3×4	3×5	3×6	3×6							
Rocket jump and star jump	107 and 108	2×4-6	2×4-6	3×4-6		3×4-6							
Split jump and scissors jump	111 and 112	2×4-6		3×4-6	3×6-8	3×6-8	3×4-6						
Prancing	120	2×4-6	2×4-6	2×4-6	2×4-6	2×4-6							
Galloping	121	3×10	3×10	3×10	3×10	2×10	2×10	2×10	2×10	2×10	2×10	2×10	2×10
Fast skipping	122	3×10	3×10	3×10	3×10	2×10	2×10	2×10	2×10	2×10	2×10	2×10	2×10
Ankle flip	125	2×4-6	3×4-6	3×4-6	3×6-8	3×6-8	3×6-8	3×6-8	3×6-8	3×6-8	2×8-10	2×8-10	2×8-10
Single-leg stair bound	127		2×4-6	2×4-6	3×6-8		2×8-10	2×8-10		2×8-10			
Lateral bound (single response)	126			2×6-8	3×6-8	3×8-10	3×8-12		3×10-12				
Alternate-leg stair bound	130		2×6-8	3×6-8	3×8-10	3×8-12	3×8-12	3×8-12					
DESIRABLES													
Overhead throw progression	68-73		2×3-6	2×3-6	2×3-6	2×3-6		2×3-6	2×3-6				
Twist toss	95			3×4-6	3×4-6	3×4-6	3×4-6	3×4-6	3×4-6	3×4-6			
Stride jump crossover	115				3×4-6	3×4-6	3×4-6	3×4-6	3×4-6	3×4-6			
Heavy bag stroke	76				3×4-6	3×4-6	3×4-6	3×4-6	3×4-6	3×4-6	3×4-6		
Horizontal swing	89				2×4-6	2×4-6	3×4-6	3×4-8	3×6-10				
Single-leg hop progression	143					2×4-6	3×4-6	3×4-6	3×6-8	3×8-10		3×8-12	
Side hop	138						2×4-6	3×4-6	3×6-8		3×6-8		3×6-8
Side hop-sprint	139								2×4-6	3×4-6	3×4-6	3×4-6	3×4-6
Lateral bound (multiple response)	126									2×4-6	3×4-6	3×4-6	3×4-6
Single-leg hop progression	143									2×3-6	3×3-6	3×3-6	3×3-6
Single-leg diagonal hop	145										2×3-6	2×3-6	3×3-6
Multiple hops to toss	83 and 86									2×3-6	2×3-6	2×3-6	2×3-6
Impact intensity			Low		Medium				High			Shock	

Table 9.17 Continuum Training for Track (Sprint, Jump, Hurdle)

PROGRAM BASICS													
Exercise	Page #	Wk 1	Wk 2	Wk 3	Wk 4	Wk 5	Wk 6	Wk 7	Wk 8	Wk 9	Wk 10	Wk 11	Wk 12
Pogo	104	3 × 10	3 × 10	3 × 10	3 × 10								
Squat jump	105	2 × 4-6	3 × 4-6	3 × 6-8									
Medicine ball over and under, medicine ball half and full twist	88, 92, and 93	3 × 3	3 × 4	3 × 5	3 × 6	3 × 6							
Rocket jump and star jump	107 and 108	2 × 4-6	2 × 4-6	3 × 4-6		3 × 4-6							
Split jump and scissors jump	111 and 112	2 × 4-6		3 × 4-6	3 × 6-8	3 × 6-8	3 × 4-6						
Prancing	120	2 × 4-6	2 × 4-6	2 × 4-6	2 × 4-6	2 × 4-6							
Galloping	121	3 × 10	3 × 10	3 × 10	3 × 10	2 × 10	2 × 10	2 × 10	2 × 10	2 × 10	2 × 10	2 × 10	2 × 10
Fast skipping	122	3 × 10	3 × 10	3 × 10	3 × 10	2 × 10	2 × 10	2 × 10	2 × 10	2 × 10	2 × 10	2 × 10	2 × 10
Ankle flip	125	2 × 4-6	3 × 4-6	3 × 4-6	3 × 6-8	3 × 6-8	3 × 6-8	3 × 6-8	3 × 6-8	3 × 6-8	2 × 8-10	2 × 8-10	2 × 8-10
Single-leg stair bound	127		2 × 4-6	2 × 4-6	3 × 6-8		2 × 8-10	2 × 8-10			2 × 8-10		
Lateral bound (single response)	126			2 × 6-8	3 × 6-8	3 × 8-10	3 × 8-12		3 × 10-12				
Alternate-leg stair bound	130		2 × 6-8	3 × 6-8	3 × 8-10	3 × 8-12	3 × 8-12	3 × 8-12					
DESIRABLES													
Knee-tuck jump	110		3 × 4-6	3 × 4-6	3 × 4-6	3 × 6-8	3 × 6-8						
Stride jump	114			3 × 4	3 × 5	3 × 6		3 × 6	3 × 6				
Alternate-leg bound	131					3 × 6-8	3 × 8-10	3 × 8-12	3 × 8-12	3 × 10+	3 × 10-12		
Double-leg slide kick	109					3 × 6-8	3 × 6-8	3 × 8-10	3 × 8-10	3 × 8-10	3 × 8-10	3 × 8-10	3 × 8-10
Single-leg hop progression	143				3 × 3	3 × 4	3 × 5	3 × 6	3 × 6	3 × 6	3 × 6	3 × 6	3 × 6
Double-leg hop progression	135 and 136					2 × 4-6	3 × 6-8	3 × 6-8	4 × 6-8	4 × 6-8	4 × 6-8	4 × 6-8	4 × 6-8
Side hop	138					2 × 4-6	2 × 4-6	3 × 4-6	3 × 4-6	3 × 6-8	3 × 6-8	3 × 6-8	3 × 6-8
Single-leg hop progression	143								2 × 3	3 × 3	3 × 3-5	3 × 5-7	3 × 6-8
Depth jump progression	117								1 × 3	1 × 4	1 × 5	1 × 7	
Combination jump and bound exercises	116-119										3 × 3	3 × 3	3 × 3
Jump decathlon	57											2 × 2	
Box bound	134											3 × 3	3 × 3
Impact intensity			Low		Medium				High			Shock	

177

Table 9.18 Continuum Training for Track and Field Throwers

Exercise	Page #	Wk 1	Wk 2	Wk 3	Wk 4	Wk 5	Wk 6	Wk 7	Wk 8	Wk 9	Wk 10	Wk 11	Wk 12
PROGRAM BASICS													
Pogo	104	3 × 10	3 × 10	3 × 10	3 × 10								
Squat jump	105	2 × 4-6	3 × 4-6	3 × 6-8									
Medicine ball over and under, medicine ball half and full twist	88, 92, and 93	3 × 3	3 × 4	3 × 5	3 × 6	3 × 6							
Rocket jump and star jump	107 and 108	2 × 4-6	2 × 4-6	3 × 4-6		3 × 4-6							
Split jump and scissors jump	111 and 112	2 × 4-6		3 × 4-6	3 × 6-8	3 × 6-8	3 × 4-6						
Prancing	120	2 × 4-6	2 × 4-6	2 × 4-6	2 × 4-6	2 × 4-6							
Galloping	121	3 × 10	3 × 10	3 × 10	3 × 10	2 × 10	2 × 10	2 × 10	2 × 10	2 × 10	2 × 10	2 × 10	2 × 10
Fast skipping	122	3 × 10	3 × 10	3 × 10	3 × 10	2 × 10	2 × 10	2 × 10	2 × 10	2 × 10	2 × 10	2 × 10	2 × 10
Ankle flip	125	2 × 4-6	3 × 4-6	3 × 4-6	3 × 6-8	3 × 6-8	3 × 6-8	3 × 6-8	3 × 6-8	3 × 6-8	2 × 8-10	2 × 8-10	2 × 8-10
Single-leg stair bound	127		2 × 4-6	2 × 4-6	3 × 6-8		2 × 8-10	2 × 8-10		2 × 8-10			
Lateral bound (single response)	126			2 × 6-8	3 × 6-8	3 × 8-10	3 × 8-12		3 × 10-12				
Alternate-leg stair bound	130		2 × 6-8	3 × 6-8	3 × 8-10	3 × 8-12	3 × 8-12	3 × 8-12					
DESIRABLES													
Incline ricochet	148	3 × 8-12	3 × 8-12	3 × 8-12	3 × 8-12	3 × 8-12	3 × 8-12						
Bar twist	94	3 × 8-12	3 × 8-12	3 × 8-12	3 × 8-12	3 × 8-12			3 × 8-12				
Twist toss progression	95	3 × 12-20		3 × 12-20	3 × 12-20		3 × 12-20	3 × 12-20					
Heavy bag thrust	75		3 × 4-6	3 × 4-6	3 × 4-6	3 × 4-6	3 × 4-6	3 × 4-6					
Heavy bag stroke	76		3 × 6-12	3 × 6-12	3 × 6-12		3 × 6-12	3 × 6-12					
Shovel toss	84		3 × 4-6	3 × 4-6	3 × 6-8	3 × 6-8			3 × 8-10	3 × 8-10			
Scoop toss progression	85				3 × 4-6	3 × 4-6	3 × 4-6			3 × 6-8	3 × 6-8	3 × 6-8	
Shovel toss progression	84			2 × 4-6		3 × 4-6	3 × 4-6	3 × 6-8	3 × 6-8		3 × 6-8		3 × 6-8
Forward throw progression	68-73			2 × 4-6	2 × 4-6	3 × 4-6	3 × 4-6	3 × 4-6		3 × 6-8	3 × 6-8	3 × 6-8	3 × 6-8
Sit-up throw progression	67			2 × 10-20	2 × 10-20		2 × 10-20		2 × 10-20	2 × 10-20	2 × 10-20	2 × 10-20	2 × 10-20
Horizontal swing	89						2 × 8-12	2 × 8-12	2 × 8-12	2 × 8-12		2 × 8-12	2 × 8-12
Floor kip	99					2 × 3-6		2 × 3-6	2 × 3-6	3 × 3-6	3 × 3-6	3 × 3-6	3 × 3-6
Impact intensity			Low		Medium				High			Shock	

Table 9.19 Continuum Training for Olympic Weightlifting

Exercise	Page #	Wk 1	Wk 2	Wk 3	Wk 4	Wk 5	Wk 6	Wk 7	Wk 8	Wk 9	Wk 10	Wk 11	Wk 12
PROGRAM BASICS													
Pogo	104	3 × 10	3 × 10	3 × 10	3 × 10								
Squat jump	105	2 × 4-6	3 × 4-6	3 × 6-8									
Medicine ball over and under, medicine ball half and full twist	88, 92, and 93	3 × 3	3 × 4	3 × 5	3 × 6	3 × 6							
Rocket jump and star jump	107 and 108	2 × 4-6	2 × 4-6	3 × 4-6		3 × 4-6							
Split jump and scissors jump	111 and 112	2 × 4-6		3 × 4-6	3 × 6-8	3 × 6-8	3 × 4-6						
Prancing	120	2 × 4-6	2 × 4-6	2 × 4-6	2 × 4-6	2 × 4-6							
Galloping	121	3 × 10	3 × 10	3 × 10	3 × 10	2 × 10	2 × 10	2 × 10	2 × 10	2 × 10	2 × 10	2 × 10	2 × 10
Fast skipping	122	3 × 10	3 × 10	3 × 10	3 × 10	2 × 10	2 × 10	2 × 10	2 × 10	2 × 10	2 × 10	2 × 10	2 × 10
Ankle flip	125	2 × 4-6	3 × 4-6	3 × 4-6	3 × 6-8	3 × 6-8	3 × 6-8	3 × 6-8	3 × 6-8	3 × 6-8	2 × 8-10	2 × 8-10	2 × 8-10
Single-leg stair bound	127		2 × 4-6	2 × 4-6	3 × 6-8		2 × 8-10	2 × 8-10			2 × 8-10		
Lateral bound (single response)	126			2 × 6-8	3 × 6-8	3 × 8-10	3 × 8-12		3 × 10-12				
Alternate-leg stair bound	130		2 × 6-8	3 × 6-8	3 × 8-10	3 × 8-12	3 × 8-12	3 × 8-12					
DESIRABLES													
Scoop toss progression	85			3 × 3-6	3 × 3-6	3 × 3-6		3 × 3-6	3 × 3-6	3 × 3-6			
Knee-tuck jump	110			3 × 3-6	3 × 3-6	3 × 3-6		3 × 3-6	3 × 3-6	3 × 3-6			
Incremental vertical hop	137				3 × 3-6	3 × 3-6	3 × 3-6		3 × 3-6	3 × 3-6	3 × 3-6		
Quick leap	116				4-8 × 1-2	4-8 × 1-2	4-8 × 1-2	4-8 × 1-2		4-8 × 1-2	4-8 × 1-2	4-8 × 1-2	4-8 × 1-2
Floor kip	99					3 × 1	3 × 1	3 × 1	3 × 1		3 × 1	3 × 1	3 × 1
Depth jump	117									4-8 × 3-6	4-8 × 3-6	4-8 × 3-6	4-8 × 3-6
Depth jump leap	119										3-6 × 3-5	3-6 × 3-5	3-6 × 3-5
Impact intensity			Low		Medium				High			Shock	

Table 9.20 Continuum Training for Wrestling

Exercise	Page #	Wk 1	Wk 2	Wk 3	Wk 4	Wk 5	Wk 6	Wk 7	Wk 8	Wk 9	Wk 10	Wk 11	Wk 12
PROGRAM BASICS													
Pogo	104	3 × 10	3 × 10	3 × 10	3 × 10								
Squat jump	105	2 × 4-6	3 × 4-6	3 × 6-8									
Medicine ball over and under, medicine ball half and full twist	88, 92, and 93	3 × 3	3 × 4	3 × 5	3 × 6	3 × 6							
Rocket jump and star jump	107 and 108	2 × 4-6	2 × 4-6	3 × 4-6		3 × 4-6							
Split jump and scissors jump	111 and 112	2 × 4-6		3 × 4-6	3 × 6-8	3 × 6-8	3 × 4-6						
Prancing	120	2 × 4-6	2 × 4-6	2 × 4-6	2 × 4-6	2 × 4-6							
Galloping	121	3 × 10	3 × 10	3 × 10	3 × 10	2 × 10	2 × 10	2 × 10	2 × 10	2 × 10	2 × 10	2 × 10	2 × 10
Fast skipping	122	3 × 10	3 × 10	3 × 10	3 × 10	2 × 10	2 × 10	2 × 10	2 × 10	2 × 10	2 × 10	2 × 10	2 × 10
Ankle flip	125	2 × 4-6	3 × 4-6	3 × 4-6	3 × 6-8	3 × 6-8	3 × 6-8	3 × 6-8	3 × 6-8	3 × 6-8	2 × 8-10	2 × 8-10	2 × 8-10
Single-leg stair bound	127		2 × 4-6	2 × 4-6	3 × 6-8		2 × 8-10	2 × 8-10		2 × 8-10			
Lateral bound (single response)	126			2 × 6-8	3 × 6-8	3 × 8-10	3 × 8-12		3 × 10-12				
Alternate-leg stair bound	130		2 × 6-8	3 × 6-8	3 × 8-10	3 × 8-12	3 × 8-12	3 × 8-12					
DESIRABLES													
Bar twist	94	3 × 8-12	3 × 8-12	3 × 8-12	3 × 8-12	3 × 8-12	3 × 8-12						
Scoop toss progression	85			3 × 8-12	3 × 8-12	3 × 8-12		3 × 8-12	3 × 8-12				
Shovel toss progression	84			3 × 12-20	3 × 12-20		3 × 12-20	3 × 12-20		3 × 12-20			
Knee-tuck jump	110				3 × 4-6	3 × 4-6	3 × 4-6	3 × 4-6	3 × 4-6	3 × 4-6			
Power skipping	123		3 × 6-12	3 × 6-12	3 × 6-12		3 × 6-12	3 × 6-12					
Single-leg stride jump	114		3 × 4-6	3 × 4-6	3 × 6-8	3 × 6-8		3 × 8-10	3 × 8-10				
Floor kip	99			2 × 6-10	2 × 6-10	2 × 6-10	3 × 6-12		3 × 6-12	3 × 6-12		3 × 6-12	
Horizontal and vertical swing	89 and 90			2 × 4-6		3 × 4-6	3 × 4-6	3 × 6-8	3 × 6-8		3 × 6-8		3 × 6-8
Leap progression	118 and 119			2 × 4-6	2 × 4-6	3 × 4-6	3 × 4-6	3 × 4-6		3 × 6-8	3 × 6-8	3 × 6-8	3 × 6-8
Side hop	138			2 × 4-6	2 × 4-6		2 × 4-6	2 × 4-6		2 × 4-6	2 × 4-6	2 × 4-6	2 × 4-6
Single-leg hop progression	143							2 × 3-6	2 × 3-6	2 × 3-6	2-3 × 3-6	3-4 × 3-6	4 × 3-6
Single-leg diagonal hop	145								2 × 3-6	3 × 3-6	3 × 3-6	3 × 3-6	3 × 3-6
Impact intensity			Low		Medium				High			Shock	

Table 9.21 Continuum Training for Aussie Football

Exercise	Page #	Wk 1	Wk 2	Wk 3	Wk 4	Wk 5	Wk 6	Wk 7	Wk 8	Wk 9	Wk 10	Wk 11	Wk 12
PROGRAM BASICS													
Pogo	104	3 × 10	3 × 10	3 × 10	3 × 10								
Squat jump	105	2 × 4-6	3 × 4-6	3 × 6-8									
Medicine ball over and under, medicine ball half and full twist	88, 92, and 93	3 × 3	3 × 4	3 × 5	3 × 6	3 × 6							
Rocket jump and star jump	107 and 108	2 × 4-6	2 × 4-6	3 × 4-6		3 × 4-6							
Split jump and scissors jump	111 and 112	2 × 4-6		3 × 4-6	3 × 6-8	3 × 6-8	3 × 4-6						
Prancing	120	2 × 4-6	2 × 4-6	2 × 4-6	2 × 4-6	2 × 4-6							
Galloping	121	3 × 10	3 × 10	3 × 10	3 × 10	2 × 10	2 × 10	2 × 10	2 × 10	2 × 10	2 × 10	2 × 10	2 × 10
Fast skipping	122	3 × 10	3 × 10	3 × 10	3 × 10	2 × 10	2 × 10	2 × 10	2 × 10	2 × 10	2 × 10	2 × 10	2 × 10
Ankle flip	125	2 × 4-6	3 × 4-6	3 × 4-6	3 × 6-8	3 × 6-8	3 × 6-8	3 × 6-8	3 × 6-8	3 × 6-8	2 × 8-10	2 × 8-10	2 × 8-10
Single-leg stair bound	127		2 × 4-6	2 × 4-6	3 × 6-8		2 × 8-10	2 × 8-10		2 × 8-10			
Lateral bound (single response)	126		2 × 6-8	3 × 6-8	3 × 8-10	3 × 8-12		3 × 10-12					
Alternate-leg stair bound	130		2 × 6-8	3 × 6-8	3 × 8-10	3 × 8-12	3 × 8-12	3 × 8-12					
DESIRABLES													
Incline ricochet	148			3 × 8-12	3 × 8-12	3 × 8-12		3 × 8-12	3 × 8-12				
Knee-tuck jump	110			3 × 4-6	3 × 4-6	3 × 4-6	3 × 4-6	3 × 4-6	3 × 4-6	3 × 4-6			
Single-leg stride jump	114				3 × 4-6	3 × 4-6	3 × 4-6	3 × 4-6	3 × 4-6	3 × 4-6			
Stride jump crossover	115					3 × 4-6	3 × 4-6	3 × 4-6	3 × 4-6	3 × 4-6	3 × 4-6		
Power skipping	123					3 × 4-6	3 × 4-6	3 × 4-6	3 × 4-8	3 × 4-8			
Alternate-leg bound	131						2 × 4-6	3 × 4-6	3 × 4-6	3 × 6-8	3 × 8-10		3 × 8-12
Incremental vertical hop	137							2 × 4-6	3 × 4-6	3 × 6-8		3 × 8-12	3 × 8-12
Side hop	138									2 × 4-6	3 × 6-8	3 × 6-8	3 × 6-10	3 × 6-10
Single-leg hop progression	143										2 × 4-6	3 × 4-6	3 × 4-6	3 × 4-6
Single-leg diagonal hop	145										2 × 3-6	3 × 3-6	3 × 3-6	3 × 3-6
Leg toss	91										2 × 3-6	4 × 3-6	4 × 3-6
Stepping two-arm overhead throw	72										2 × 3-6	4 × 3-6	4 × 3-6
Impact intensity			Low		Medium				High			Shock	

MOUNTAIN AND RIVER ROUTINES

Once athletes have performed the program basics and then the specific desirable dozen exercises for their sport or activity, they can perform certain routines on certain days either weekly or biweekly. These multiple plyometric routines of jumps, bounds, hops, and throws are advanced based on dosages and intensities, but they do not necessarily have to be high or shock stress.

The mountain and river routines fit best into the advanced or competitive phase of training. (We call these routines mountains and rivers for convenience in referring to them by name. Athletes might prefer to personalize them, perhaps naming them after their favorite athletes. Coaches might name them after former favorite students.) In any case, athletes should probably not advance to the mountain and river routines until they have accomplished all the progressions initially, rehabilitatively, and transitionally (from the end of the competitive season into the next preparatory season). As discussed in chapter 10, athletes can progress into and out of levels of stretch–shortening cycle training during phases of the precompetitive and competitive periods in several ways. One way to do this is to cycle variations of the mountain and river routines into particular competitive training periods.

Athletes and coaches can set up their own series of mountains and rivers (see table 9.22) based on athletes' accomplishments and needs and the goals of the competitive training period.

Table 9.22 Mountain and River Plyometric Routines

MOUNTAIN ROUTINES		
Mt. McKinley Horizontal work: 1. Prancing (p. 120) 2. Galloping (p. 121) 3. Ankle flip (p. 125) 4. Alternate-leg bound (p. 131) 5. Extended skipping (p. 124) 6. Box bound (p. 134)	The Matterhorn Vertical work: 1. Rocket jump and star jump (pp. 107 and 108) 2. Knee-tuck jump (p. 110) 3. Split jump and scissors jump (pp. 111 and 112) 4. Power skipping (p. 123) 5. Box jump (p. 106) 6. Depth jump (p. 117)	Mt. Fuji Combinations: 1. Single-leg slide kick (p. 142) 2. Double-leg speed hop (p. 136) 3. Single-leg hop (p. 143) 4. Extended skipping (p. 124) 5. Box skip (p. 133) 6. Box bound (p. 134)
Mt. Everest Stairs: 1. Double-leg incline bound (p. 128) 2. Power skipping (p. 123) 3. Single-leg stair bound (p. 127) 4. Lateral bound (p. 126) 5. Alternate-leg bound (p. 131) 6. Incline ricochet (p. 148)	Mt. Olympus Lateral: 1. Lateral bound (p. 126) 2. Side hop (p. 138) 3. Incremental vertical hop (p. 137) 4. Alternate-leg diagonal bound (p. 132) 5. Single-leg diagonal hop (p. 145) 6. Single-leg lateral hop (p. 146)	
RIVER ROUTINES		
Missouri River Rotational: 1. Medicine ball half twist (p. 92) 2. Medicine ball full twist (p. 93) 3. Bar twist (p. 94) 4. Horizontal swing (p. 89) 5. Twist toss (p. 95) 6. Heavy bag thrust and heavy bag stroke (pp. 75 and 76)	Columbia River Tossing: 1. Shovel toss (p. 84) 2. Scoop toss (p. 85) 3. Vertical swing (p. 90) 4. Medicine ball chest pass (p. 65) 5. Multiple hops to underhand toss (p. 86) 6. Backward hops to underhand toss (p. 86)	Mississippi River Throwing: 1. Sit-up throw (p. 67) 2. Kneeling two-arm overhead throw (p. 70) 3. Standing or stepping throw (pp. 71 or 72) 4. Scoop toss (p. 85) 5. Multiple hops to overhead throw (p. 83) 6. Catch and overhead throw (p. 73)

SPORT- AND EVENT-SPECIFIC ROUTINES

The routines in table 9.23 can be used to enhance specific aspects of events that occur in many of the aforementioned sports.

Table 9.23   Sport- and Event-Specific Plyometric Routines

Starting	Accelerating	Stopping (decelerating)
1. Squat jump (p. 105)	1. Prancing (p. 120)	1. Depth jump (p. 117)
2. Quick leap (p. 116)	2. Galloping (p. 121)	2. Quick leap (p. 116)
3. Double-leg slide kick (p. 109)	3. Ankle flip (p. 125)	3. Depth leap (p. 118)
4. Knee-tuck jump (p. 110)	4. Alternate-leg bound (p. 131)	4. Extended skipping (p. 124)
5. Split jump (p. 111)	5. Fast skipping (p. 122)	5. Multiple hops to overhead throw (p. 83)
6. Medicine ball chest pass (p. 65)	6. Power skipping (p. 123)	6. Multiple hops to chest push (p. 83; use chest push instead of overhead throw)
	7. Extended skipping (p. 124)	
	8. Box bound (p. 134)	
Speeding	Changing	
1. Pogo (p. 104)	1. Side hop (p. 138)	
2. Single-leg pogo (p. 141)	2. Incremental vertical hop (p. 137)	
3. Stride jump progression (p. 114)	3. Lateral bound (p. 126)	
4. Decline hop (p. 147)	4. Alternate-leg diagonal bound (p. 132)	
5. Double-leg hop (p. 135)	5.Single-leg diagonal hop (p. 145)	
6. Single-leg hop (p. 143)	6. Single-leg lateral hop (p. 146)	

Season-Long Power Maintenance

Training is organized instruction that is directed within a time framework toward specific goals. The final task we undertake in this book is to look at the stretch–shortening cycle in a broad sense, attempting to see as big a picture as possible. Using terms associated with endurance training, muscular hypertrophy training (bodybuilding), and absolute strength training has often been taboo in plyometrics, simply because they tend to be on the other end of the training spectrum from explosion, impulsion, and reaction. When we refer to explosive power training, many of us, purists perhaps, still defend the true intentions of plyometric (i.e., shock-style) training, in which long, slow overdosages intended to produce size or cardiorespiratory improvements do not often fit. However, the stretch–shortening cycle can still be a valuable tool to complement those training areas.

Long-term planning and promotion are essential to mastering training and performance, not to mention a sport itself. Program design—encompassing all facets of strength, speed, agility, and plyometric training; the stretch–shortening cycle; and evaluation—presents many questions, some of which can be answered easily, some of which require research to answer, and others of which can only be answered by trial, error, retrial, and the passage of time.

At some point, progressions (and progress!) take us from development to refinement. Refining power is not ceasing the development process. Rather, it is an elite approach to the transitional phase of skill mastery, the extreme specificity of power as it applies to the movement, athlete, activity, and sport.

The concept of planned performance training, or periodization as it is known to many, can be explained using the following analogy. If a single coach and one or two athletes need to travel from Boston to Atlanta, the overall planning can be fairly simple. Deciding what vehicle to use and what route to take is easy because the group is small. They may not have to plan out their stops, meal breaks, and bathroom breaks. They simply need to choose the best route and make small adjustments so that they keep traveling on that route. On the other hand, if a coach or coaching staff and 35 or 40 athletes need to get from Boston to Atlanta, a plan becomes much more important. What form of transportation is best— a plane, train, bus, or hot air balloon? What is best for the needs of the group as a whole? If they choose ground travel, when and where will they stop? Will it be every time someone is hungry or needs to use facilities? Or will there be planned stops for the entire team? What if there is a detour or delay? Does the group adjust for certain people, or for the entire group? How often?

These kinds of decisions are the reason for periodic planned performance protocols, or periodization. These decisions are not, nor should they ever be, written in stone (i.e., unchangeable). Just like the traveling party of three, which can adjust easily to the needs of one, the party of 40 needs to adjust as well, occasionally to the needs of one or two. If the plan is flexible and factors in possible disasters, delays, and dilemmas, then the group can travel optimally to the destination. Similarly, progressions in training address the fact that some people will not be able to travel as quickly and easily down each planned route as others might. They can still train and develop optimally, though, just at a different pace. And they are still en route to the destination, often with fewer off-route disasters because of the proper progressive approach.

YEAR-ROUND PERFORMANCE TRAINING

Developing the goals of a training program involves establishing the peak, or final competitions, and working backward from that point. Whether the peak is a single competitive situation (e.g., the Tour de France), a portion of a season (state playoffs), or a multipeaking competition (e.g., national, Pan-American, world, or Olympic championships), each goal can be addressed by using the evaluation continuums and the program hierarchy to map the route of the stretch–shortening cycle training in each period of the yearly plan (see figure 10.1).

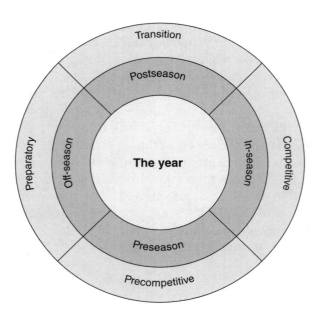

Figure 10.1 The yearly overview.

Just as athletes progress and cycle through a training format for stretch–shortening cycle, or plyometric, methodology, they can also progress and cycle through phases, periods, and years—in both the short term and the long term. Moreover, periods can be planned for both individuals and teams. The principle of multilateral periodization (i.e., involving several systems of training), from general to specific training, involves exposing younger athletes to mixed or multidirectional training as mentioned in the previous discussion of hierarchy concepts. Advanced athletes, those who have developed high levels of core, relative, and dynamic strength, can use prioritized or unidirectional (i.e., highly specific) training. In some situations, athletes perform no conventional strength training in a microcycle dominated by elastic–reactive training. In all cases, repetitions, sets, and rest periods should reflect training objectives.

Periods

Training year period objectives differ based on the training program. For some athletes, periods merely reflect a change of season: in-season (competitive), postseason (regenerative), off-season (general preparatory), and preseason (special preparatory). For multisport athletes and those who perform only in-season training, periods have different objectives. In many situations, the competitive period is a time to back off ardent stretch–shortening cycle and plyometric drills other than those designed to meet competition objectives (e.g., specific jumping, sprinting, and change-of-direction drills). Developing power takes a back seat to refining speed skills.

However, these athletes may miss all opportunities for basic and special development. Applying methodologies within the power hierarchy can be helpful in both cases. The stretch–shortening cycle is evident in many forms of preparatory, or technical, work, as well as in developmental loading and specific transitional work (see figure 10.2a for those new to plyometrics and 10.2b for those experienced in explosive power). The program planner can prioritize the training cycles within the competitive period, formulating a miniature version of the combination of periods that mimic the progressive nature of the big picture.

In summary, training periods are steps toward peak performance. Table 10.1 presents a list of periods and their objectives.

Phases

As Bompa (1983) suggested, each period has cycled phases that generate the advancement to specific objectives for each training season. Recommendations to continue plyometric training over several months are not uncommon. Indeed, we believe that athletes can adhere to a continuous, year-round approach. Some believe that plyometric drills should be used only for three or four weeks of training microcycles. This may come from some practitioners' notion of a limited ability to train certain speed segments. Zanon (1989), for example, recommended a cyclic oscillatory trend of increased plyometric use for 10 days and then decreased use for 10 days, regulated over a three-week cycle. When using a progressive system of stress-continuum plyometrics, we believe that elastic–reactive movements can be used throughout the training phase, at least until major competitive peaking cycles occur. As a result of proprioceptive progress, this can offer the advantage of year-round SSC and plyometric attention. Periodic planning of the progressive

Preparation		Evaluation	
Transition	Preparatory	Precompetitive	Competitive
Regeneration	Technical enhancement	Developmental refinement	Specific maintenance
Program basics	Program basics	Desirable dozens	Tapered basics
First 12 weeks	Repeat 12 weeks	12-week segment	Technical and preparational
0-2 years training ages from beginner to intermediate			

a

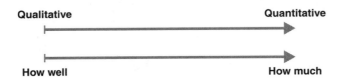

Qualitative   Quantitative

How well   How much

Preparation		Evaluation	
Transition	Preparatory	Precompetitive	Competitive
Regeneration	Technical enhancement	Developmental refinement	Specific maintenance
Program basics	Program basics	Specific development	Tapered preparational and technical work
Continuum work	Continuum work	Work cycles	
Simple progressions	More specific progressions	Mountains and rivers	Continuum revisited
2+ years of training age intermediate to advanced stages			

b

Figure 10.2 Use of the stretch–shortening cycle in *(a)* early training periodization and *(b)* advanced periodization.

methods of strength, speed, and elastic training is presented in figure 10.3 (Bompa 1983 and Radcliffe 1998).

At the end of the chapter we offer samples of procedures through a period of training phases. The charts of the annual plans can be rotated to fit numerous activities and their objectives. Athletes should apply progressive patterns through the stretch–shortening cycle and plyometric forms of training and consider their suitability in the hierarchy of power development. They can then emphasize different areas of stretch–shortening cycle development, be it a dynamic warm-up; technical, developmental, or specific mobility work during training workouts; or competitive practices in each phase. To achieve sport-specific goals, athletes must determine how much stretch–shortening cycle training is needed and where. They can then analyze their performance in the specific training to decide whether to continue at the same dosages, increase volumes, taper dosages, or cease the training for specific competitive reasons.

Table 10.1 Training Period Objectives

Period	Type of period	Objectives
Postseason	Transitional period	• Recovering, restoring, and regenerating from the previous competitive season • Developing or rehabilitating work capacity in strength, acceleration, and mobility • Making technical readjustments and refinements
Off-season	Preparatory period	• Progressively developing work capacities in strength, speed, and agility • Technically advancing and evaluating performance in competitive situations
Preseason	Precompetitive period	• Refining specific work capacities in strength, speed, and agility with conversions to specific power and speed endurance • Specifically advancing performance in the competitive situation • Tapering the training model • Heightening the performance methodologies
In-season	Competitive period	• Expanding the competition experience • Maintaining development of the power and specific speed and speed-endurance skills, which may mean moving back to early and simple plyometric progressions that can be included in warm-up or posttraining sessions, thereby reducing the overall work time and load • Advancing specific techniques • Preparing for competition climax • Achieving an a optimal performance at the finish of the competition period

Strength training phases	Preparational		Evaluative/competitive	
	Build-up prep work	Maximum work	Conversion to specifics	Maintenance

Speed training phases	Preparational		Evaluative/competitive	
	Acceleration	Speed	Speed endurance	Specific maintenance

Elastic training phases	Preparational		Evaluative/competitive	
	Begin progressions jump toss	Bound hop throw	Combos and shock methods	Maintenance routines

• A blend of guidelines that progress equally and efficiently through the training and competing phases

• Progressions that graduate in technique complexity, impact intensity, and competition-specific volumes and durations

Figure 10.3 Periodic phases of training methodologies.

For our purposes, and the efficiency of the weekly workload, we like to use 21- to 28-day training cycles (three to four weeks). Our most common practice is to use a four-week block of 21 days of progressive development and an off-loading or evaluation week (see figure 10.4).

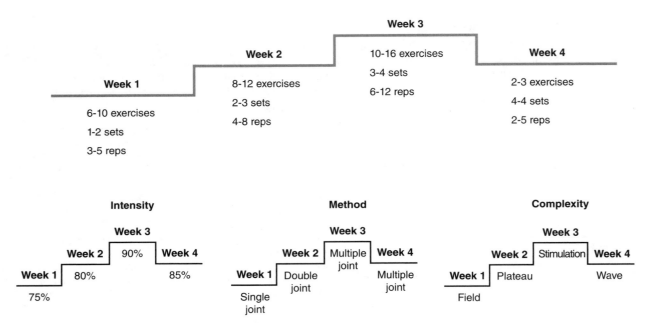

Figure 10.4   Four-week training cycles that progress in volume, intensity, method, complexity, or total accumulated workload for the first three weeks, then are off-loaded during the fourth week. Jumping or throwing tests can be used to evaluate progress either at the beginning of specified weeks or during the fourth week.

SEASONAL CONDITIONING

A power hierarchy (see figure 10.5) is useful in planning the types and magnitudes of SSC work within the scope of a program. As athletes move through the training phases, they can also move through the training methods within the structure of the power hierarchy.

As the power hierarchy and the workout methods within it show, a great deal of stretch–shortening cycle work can be accomplished throughout the entire scope of the training. Throughout the stages of the program, each level has a definite place in the workout's power hierarchy. For example, the progression of pogo, prancing, galloping, and so on, which was the main focus of the plyometric and loading workout at the beginning of the program, can eventually become part of the technical period (form running) and even the preparatory period (dynamic warm-up). This provides constant attention to developing biomechanical skills in their parts while progressing to the more complex and intense forms of stretch–shortening cycle training as a whole. Often, planners wonder when to emphasize plyometric drills versus weight training, and vice versa. When working within the context of the hierarchy and the progressions we provide, the main concern is meeting the objectives of the particular cycle in the training phase.

Each workout, whether performed in a weight room, on a court, or on a field, can adhere to the methodologies. The methodologies can be applied to a preparatory session (dynamic and static flexibility), a technical session (form running and lifting movements), a developmental session (all forms of loading, extended durations, and speeds), or a transitional mobility session (changes of direction, high-speed executions).

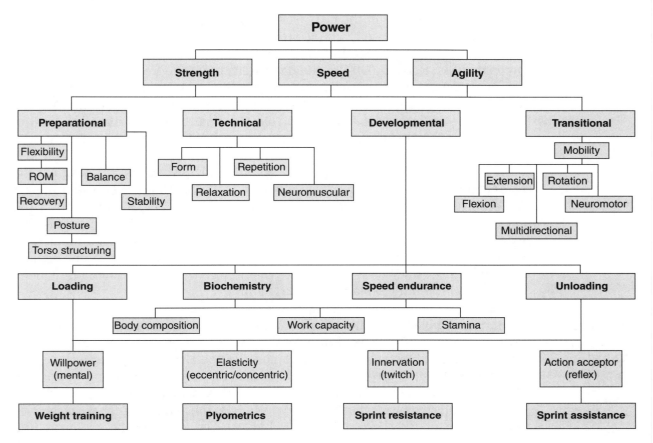

Figure 10.5 Power hierarchy.

If weight training includes postural and dynamic forms of lifting (which we think it should), the timing of the training method merely depends on the placement of the workout session. Some trainers and sport scientists suggest that training sessions include a warm-up and dynamic work, followed by strength work and speed work, and end with a cool-down. This is one way, as is the power hierarchy method, of establishing when to emphasize the degree of workload. We need to make several points about using stretch–shortening cycle training, whether the design is for plyometrics, Olympic lifting, speed work, or agility and mobility. We consider all these training types to be stretch–shortening cycle training and see it, as mentioned in chapter 1 with certain goals and objectives for dynamic force development, as an all-encompassing entity.

INDIVIDUALIZING THE TRAINING PROGRAM

For best results, plyometric training programs should be individualized. Following an evaluation, participants should be trained in the basics and observed performing some exercises. This should provide a good idea of what they are capable of and how fast they may progress. Despite continuing research in the area of optimal training loads, as in so many other areas of sport training, individualizing the stretch–shortening cycle training program is more of an art than a science.

You may notice that in the progressive development of the stretch–shortening cycle, or in a plyometric training program, some parts of the early drills and exercises that are designed to foster correct technical and developmentally safe performances do not adhere to the definitions of elastic, reactive, or plyometric exercise training. If the objectives of the overall power development program are sincere, then we must get beyond the discrepancies of single response, responses with pause, and two-foot takeoffs so that the final outcome—the elite level of progression—is truly explosive, impulsive, elastic–reactive, plyometric, and impressive.

As Siff and Verkhoshansky (1996) pointed out, plyometric training can be arranged in many categories. One example is the distinction between impact (an eccentric movement that ends in contact with a surface) and nonimpact (no surface contact ending stretch–shortening cycle movements). Distinctions also exist between maximal exercises (producing rebound tensions and impulses of the highest intensities) and submaximal exercises (exhibiting lesser impulses and lower intensities and being less complex in execution). These distinctions fit along the stress continuum explained in chapter 3.

Many movements may be preparatory, or supplemental, before progressing to more classic plyometric movements. Again, understanding the concepts of the training and the proper lead-up progressions and evaluating execution before advancing are important to the development of the plyometric program.

Before beginning stretch–shortening cycle and plyometric training, athletes should fully understand the program in which they want to incorporate it. This is best accomplished by establishing objectives from the beginning. These objectives help athletes define the training style, balance and progress the exercises, and apply training principles throughout the program.

Here are examples of objectives for establishing a program:

1. Develop a well-balanced, well-rounded, progressive training program.
2. Include the stretch–shortening cycle in all applications of basic training development (e.g., preparatory, technical, developmental, and transitional).
3. Individualize the program to safely help participants progress from beginners to advanced or elite performers.
4. Create a system for evaluating participants and the program.

The best training programs use proper progressions. By always checking the posture, balance, stability, and flexibility of each athlete throughout the program, coaches gather a great deal of information that can help them apply proper dosages and load intensities.

References

Preface

Zanon, S. 1989. Plyometrics: Past and present. *New Studies in Athletics* 4 (1): 7-17.

Chapter 1

Aoki, H., R. Tsukahara, and K. Yabe. 1989. Effects of pre-motion electromyographic silent period on dynamic force exertion during a rapid ballistic movement in man. *European Journal of Applied Physiology* 58(4): 426-432.

Bosch, F., and R. Klomp. 2005. *Running: Biomechanics and exercise physiology applied to practice.* London: Livingstone.

Bosco, C., and P.V. Komi. 1979. Mechanical characteristics and fiber composition of human leg extensor muscles. *European Journal of Applied Physiology* 41: 275-284.

Cavagna, G.A. 1977. Storage and utilization of elastic energy in skeletal muscle. *Exercise and Sports Science Review* 5:89-129.

Curwin, S., and W.D. Stanish. 1984. *Tendinitis: Its etiology and treatment.* Lexington, MA: Collamore Press.

Ebbeling, C.B., and P.M. Clarkson. 1990. Muscle adaptation prior to recovery following eccentric exercise. *European Journal of Applied Physiology* 60(1): 26-31.

Frid'en, J. 1984. Changes in human skeletal muscle induced by long term eccentric exercise. *Cell Tissue Research* 236(2): 365-372.

Fritz, V.K., and W.T. Stauber. 1988. Characterization of muscles injured by forced lengthening II: Proteoglycans. *Medicine and Science in Sports and Exercise* 20(4): 354-361.

Gambetta, V. November 1986. Velocity of shortening as an explanation for the training effect of plyometric training. Second Allerton Symposium, G. Winkler (chair), Track and Field Training, Monticello, IL.

Hewitt T.E., G.D. Myer, K.R. Ford, and J.R. Slautrbeck. 2006. Preparticipation physical examination using a box drop vertical jump test in young athletes: The effects of puberty and sex. *Clinical Journal of Sport Medicine* 16(4):298-304.

Hewitt, T.E., et al. 1999. The effect of neuromuscular training on the incidence of knee injury in female athletes: A prospective study. *American Journal of Sports Medicine.* 27(6) 699-706.

Hewitt, T.E., G.D. Myer, K.R. Ford, et al. 2005. Biomechanical measures of neuromuscular control and valgus loading of the knee predict anterior cruciate ligament injury risk in female athletes: a prospective study. *American Journal of Sports Medicine.* 33(4):492-501.

Hill, A.V. 1950. The series elastic component of muscle (summary). Proceedings of the Royal Society of London (Biology) 137: 273-280.

King, I. 1993. Plyometric training: In perspective. Parts 1 and 2. *Science Periodical on Research and Technology in Sport 13* (5 and 6).

Komi, P.V. 1973. Measurement of the force-velocity relationship in human muscle under concentric and eccentric contractions. *Medicine and Sport: Biomechanics* III 8: 224-229.

Komi, P.V. 1984a. Biomechanics and neuromuscular performance. *Medicine and Science in Sport and Exercise* 16: 26-28.

Komi, P.V. 1984b. Physiological and biomechanical correlates of muscle function: Effects of muscle structure and stretch-shortening cycle on force and speed. In *Exercise and sports science reviews* 12: 81-121, edited by R.L. Terjung.

Komi, P.V. 1986. The stretch-shortening cycle and human power output. In *Human muscle power*, edited by N.L. Jones, N. McCartney, and A. McComas.

Matveyev, L. 1977. *Fundamentals of sports training.* Moscow: Progress.

McArdle, W., F.I. Katch, and V.L. Katch. 1981. *Exercise physiology, energy, nutrition and human performance.* Philadelphia: Lea & Febiger.

Onate J, N. Cortes, C. Welch, and B.L. Van Lunen. 2010. Expert versus novice interrater reliability and criterion validity of the landing error scoring system. *Journal of Sport Rehabilitation* 19(1):41-56.

Padua D.A., M.C. Boling, L.J. DiStefano, J.A. Onate, A.I. Beutler, and S.W. Marshall. 2011. Reliability of the Landing Error Scoring System-real time: A clinical assessment tool of jump-landing biomechanics. *Journal of Sport Rehabilitation* 20:145-156.

Padua, D.A., S.W. Marshall, M.C. Boling, C.A. Thigpen, W.E. Garrett Jr., and A.I. Beutler. 2009. The Landing Error Scoring System (LESS) is a valid and reliable clinical assessment tool of jump-landing biomechanics: The JUMP-ACL study. *American Journal of Sports Medicine* 37:1996-2002

Schmidtbleicher, D. 1992. Training for power events. In *Strength and Power for Sports.* P. Komi (editor). Hoboken, NJ: Blackwell (18):382-385

Siff, M., and Y. Verkhoshansky. 1996. *Supertraining: Special strength training for sporting excellence.* 2d ed. Pittsburgh: Sports Support Syndicate.

Stauber, W. 1989. Eccentric action of muscles: Physiology, injury, and adaptation. *Exercise and Sport Science Reviews* 17: 157-185.

Weyand, P.G., D.B. Sternlight, M.J. Bellizzi, and S. Wright. 2000. Faster top running speeds are achieved with greater forces not more rapid leg movements. *Journal of Applied Physiology* 89(5)1991-1999.

Wilson, G.J., R.U. Newton, A.J. Murphy, and B.J. Humphries. 1993. The optimal training load for the development of dynamic athletic performance. *Medicine and Science in Sports and Exercise* 25(11): 1279-1286.

Winkler, G. Reflections and new direction. October 2009. 19th NACACTFCA International Athletic Congress, San Juan, Puerto Rico.

Zatsiorsky, V.M. 1995. *Science and practice of strength training.* Champaign, IL: Human Kinetics.

Chapter 2

Cramer, J.T., T.J. Housh, J.P. Weis, G.O. Johnson, J.W. Coburn, and T.W. Beck 2005. The acute effects of static stretch on peak torque, mean power output, electromyography and mechanomyography. *European Journal of Applied Physiology* 93(5-6) 530-539.

Erro, M.C. 1995. Erroisms. Enterprise High School football history. enterprisehornets.com.

Gambetta, V. 1992. Building and rebuilding the athlete. (DVD series of seminars.) www.functionalpathtrainingblog.com/2013/02/building-rebuilding-the-athlete-seminar-dvds.html.

Shrier, I. 2004 Does stretching improve performance? A systematic and critical review of the literature. *Clinical Journal of Sport Medicine* 14(5): 267-273.

Young, W., and D. Behm. 2002. Should static stretching be used during a warm-up for strength and power activities? *NSCA Journal* (24) 6:33-37.

Chapter 3

Adams, T.M. 1984. An investigation of selected plyometric training exercises on muscular leg strength and power. *Track and Field Quarterly Review* 84 (4): 36-39.

Bobbert, M.F., M. Mackey, D. Schinkelshoek, P. Huijing, and G. van Ingen Schenau. 1986. Biomechanical analysis of drop and countermovement jumps. *European Journal of Applied Physiology* 54: 566-573.

Bobbert, M.F., P.A. Huijing, and G.J. van Ingen Schenau. 1987a. Drop jumping I: The influence of jumping technique on the biomechanics of jumping. *Medicine and Science in Sports and Exercise* 19: 332-338.

Bobbert, M.F., P.A. Huijing, and G.J. van Ingen Schenau. 1987b. Drop jumping II: The influence of drop heights on the biomechanics of drop jumping. *Medicine and Science in Sports and Exercise* 19: 339-346.

Bompa, T. 1993. *Periodization of strength, the new wave in strength training.* Toronto: Veritas.

Bosco C., and P.V. Komi. 1981. Potentiation of the mechanical behavior of the human skeletal muscle through prestretching. *Acta Physiologica Scandinavia* 106: 467-472.

Bosco C., and P.V. Komi. 1981. Potentiation of the mechanical behavior of the human skeletal muscle through prestretching. *Acta Physiologica Scandinavia* 106: 467-472.

Bosco, C. 1982. Physiological considerations of strength and explosive power and jumping drills (plyometric exercise). Conference proceedings on planning for elite performance (pp. 27-37). Ottawa, ON: Canadian Track and Field Association.

Bosco, C., and P.V. Komi. 1979. Mechanical characteristics and fiber composition of human leg extensor muscles. *European Journal of Applied Physiology* 41: 275-284.

Bosco, C., and P.V. Komi. 1979. Mechanical characteristics and fiber composition of human leg extensor muscles. *European Journal of Applied Physiology* 41: 275-284.

Bosco, C., and P.V. Komi. 1982. Muscle elasticity in athletes. In *Exercise and sport biology* (pp. 109-117), edited by P.V. Komi. Champaign, IL: International Series on Sports Sciences.

Clutch, D., M. Wilton, C. McGowan, and G.R. Bryce. 1983. The effects of depth jumps and weight training on leg strength and vertical jump. *Research Quarterly for Exercise and Sport* 54:5-10.

Gambetta, V., R. Rogers, R. Fields, D. Semenick, and J. Radcliffe. 1986. NSCA plyometric videotape symposium, Lincoln, NE.

Hakkinen, K., M. Alen, and P.V. Komi. 1985. Changes in isometric force- and relaxation-time, electromyographic and muscle fiber characteristics of human skeletal muscle during strength training and detraining. *Acta Physiologica* Scandinavia 125: 573-585.

Jacoby, E., and B. Fraley. 1995. *Complete book of jumps.* Champaign, IL: Human Kinetics.

Komi, P.V., and C. Bosco. 1978. Utilization of stored elastic energy in leg extensor muscles by men and women. *Medicine and Science in Sports* 10: 261-265.

Radcliffe, J., and L. Osternig. 1995. Effects on performance of variable eccentric loads during depth jumps. *Journal of Sport Rehabilitation* 4: 31-41.

Scoles, G. 1978. Depth jumping! Does it really work? *The Athletic Journal* 58(5): 48-49, 74-75.

Siff, M., and Y. Verkhoshansky. 1996. *Supertraining: Special strength training for sporting excellence.* 2d ed. Pittsburgh: Sports Support Syndicate.

Verkhoshansky, Y. 1967. Are depth jumps useful? *Track & Field* 12:9.

Verkhoshansky, Y. 1968. Are depth jumps useful? *Yessis Review of Soviet Physical Education and Sports* 3:75-78.

Verkhoshansky, Y., and V. Tatyan. 1973. Speed-strength preparation of future champions. *Legkaya Atletica* 2: 12-13.

Viitasalo, J.T., and Bosco, C. 1982. Electromechanical behaviour of human muscles in vertical jumps. *European Journal of Applied Physiology* 48: 253-261.

Chapter 4

Bosco C., and P.V. Komi. 1981. Potentiation of the mechanical behavior of the human skeletal muscle through prestretching. *Acta Physiologica Scandinavia* 106: 467-472.

Costello, F. 1984. Using weight training and plyometrics to increase explosive power for football. *National Strength and Conditioning Association Journal* 6(2): 22-25.

Hewitt, T.E., G.D. Myer, and K.R. Ford et al. 2005. Biomechanical measures of neuromuscular control and valgus loading of the knee predict anterior cruciate ligament injury risk in female athletes: A prospective study. *American Journal of Sports Medicine* 33(4):492-501.

Hewitt, T.E., G.D. Myer, K.R. Ford, and J.R. Slautrbeck. 2006. Preparticipation physical examination using a box drop vertical jump test in young athletes: The effects of puberty and sex. *Clinical Journal of Sports Medicine* 16(4):298-304.

McFarlane, B. 1982. Jumping exercises. *Track and Field Quarterly Review* 82(4): 54-55.

Padua, D.A., S.W. Marshall, M.C. Boling, C.A. Thigpen, W.E. Garrett Jr., and A.I. Beutler. 2009. The Landing Error Scoring System (LESS) is a valid and reliable clinical assessment tool of jump-landing biomechanics: The JUMP-ACL study. *American Journal of Sports Medicine* 37:1996-2002.

Paish, W. 1968. The jumps decathlon tables. In D.C.V. Watts, *The long jump*. London: Amateur Athletic Association.

Radcliffe, J., and L. Osternig. 1995. Effects on performance of variable eccentric loads during depth jumps. *Journal of Sport Rehabilitation* 4: 31-41.

Radcliffe, J., and L. Osternig. 1995. Effects on performance of variable eccentric loads during depth jumps. *Journal of Sport Rehabilitation* 4: 31-41.

Valik, B. 1966. Strength preparation of young track and fielders. Physical Culture in School 4: 28. In *Yessis Translation Review* (1967) 2: 56-60.

Watts, D.C.V. *The long jump*. London: Amateur Athletic Association.

Chapter 8

Chu, D.A. 1996. Explosive power and strength: Complex training for maximum results. Champaign, IL: Human Kinetics.

Comyns, T.M., A.J. Harrison, L.K. Hennessy, and R.L. Jensen. 2006. The optimal complex training rest interval for athletes from anaerobic sports. *Journal of Strength and Conditioning Research* 20(3), 471-476.

Duthie, G.M., W.B. Young, and D.A. Aitken 2002. The acute effects of heavy loads on jump squat performance: An evaluation of the complex and contrast methods of power development. *Journal of Strength and Conditioning Research* 16:530-538.

Ebben, W.P. 2002. Complex training: A brief review. *Journal of Sports Science and Medicine* 2:42-46.

Ebben, W.P., and D.O. Blackard. 1997. Complex training with combined explosive weight training and plyometric exercises. *Olympic Coach* 7(4):11-12

Fees, M.A. January 1997. Complex training. *Athletic Therapy Today* 18.

Fleck, S.J., and Kontor, K. 1986. Complex training. *NSCA Journal* 8(5), 66-68.

French, D.N., W.J. Kraemer, and C.B. Cooke. 2003. Changes in dynamic exercise performance following a sequence of preconditioning isometric muscle actions. *Journal of Strength and Conditioning Research* 17:678-685.

Gambetta, V., and J Radcliffe. 1989. Delineations. B.C. Coaching Conference Keys to Coaching, Vancouver.

Harris, N.K., J.B. Cronin, W.G. Hopkins, and K.T. Hansen. 2000. Squat jump training at maximal power loads vs. heavy loads: Effects on sprint ability. *Journal of Strength and Conditioning Research* 22(6), 1742-1749.

Jones, P., and Lees, A. 2003. A biomechanical analysis of the acute effects of complex training using lower limb exercises. *Journal of Strength and Conditioning Research* 17(4), 694-700.

MacDonald, C.J., H.S. Lamont, J.C. Garner, and K. Jackson. 2013. A comparison of the effects of six week of traditional resistance training, plyometric training, and complex training on measures of power. *Journal of Strength and Conditioning Research* 26(2):422-31.

Verkhoshansky, N. 1966. Perspectives in the improvement of speed-strength preparation of jumpers. *Track and Field* 9:11-12.

Chapter 10

Adams, T.M. 1984. An investigation of selected plyometric training exercises on muscular leg strength and power. *Track and Field Quarterly Review* 84(4): 36-39.

Bobbert, M.F., M. Mackey, D. Schinkelshoek, P. Huijing, and G. van Ingen Schenau. 1986. Biomechanical analysis of drop and countermovement jumps. *European Journal of Applied Physiology* 54: 566-573.

Bobbert, M.F., P.A. Huijing, and G.J. van Ingen Schenau. 1987a. Drop jumping I: The influence of jumping technique on the biomechanics of jumping. *Medicine and Science in Sports and Exercise* 19: 332-338.

Bobbert, M.F., P.A. Huijing, and G.J. van Ingen Schenau. 1987b. Drop jumping II: The influence of drop heights on the biomechanics of drop jumping. *Medicine and Science in Sports and Exercise* 19: 339-346.

Bompa, T. 1983. *Theory and methodology of training, the key to athletic performance.* Dubuque, IA: Kendall/Hunt.

Bompa, T. 1993. Periodization of strength, the new wave in strength training. Toronto: Veritas.

Bosco C., and P.V. Komi. 1981. Potentiation of the mechanical behavior of the human skeletal muscle through prestretching. Acta Physiologica Scandinavia 106: 467-472.

Bosco, C., and P.V. Komi. 1979. Mechanical characteristics and fiber composition of human leg extensor muscles. *European Journal of Applied Physiology* 41: 275-284.

Bosco, C., and P.V. Komi. 1979. Mechanical characteristics and fiber composition of human leg extensor muscles. *European Journal of Applied Physiology* 41: 275-284.

Bosco, C., and P.V. Komi. 1982. Muscle elasticity in athletes. In *Exercise and sport biology*, edited by P.V. Komi. Champaign, IL: International Series on Sports Sciences.

Bosco, C., and P.V. Komi. 1982. Muscle elasticity in athletes. In *Exercise and sport biology*, edited by P.V. Komi. Champaign, IL: International Series on Sports Sciences.

Clutch, D., M. Wilton, C. McGowan, and G.R. Bryce. 1983. The effects of depth jumps and weight training on leg strength and vertical jump. *Research Quarterly for Exercise and Sport* 54:5-10.

Curwin, S., and W.D. Stanish. 1984. *Tendinitis: Its etiology and treatment.* Lexington, MA: Collamore Press.

Hakkinen, K., M. Alen, and P.V. Komi. 1985. Changes in isometric force- and relaxation-time, electromyographic and muscle fiber characteristics of human skeletal muscle during strength training and detraining. *Acta Physiologica Scandinavia* 125: 573-585.

Komi, P.V., and C. Bosco. 1978. Utilization of stored elastic energy in leg extensor muscles by men and women. *Medicine and Science in Sports* 10: 261-265.

Radcliffe, J., and L. Osternig. 1995. Effects on performance of variable eccentric loads during depth jumps. *Journal of Sport Rehabilitation* 4: 31-41.

Radcliffe, J.C., and R.C. Farentinos 1998. *High-powered plyometrics.* Champaign, IL: Human Kinetics.

Radcliffe, J.C., and R.C. Farentinos. 1985. Plyometrics explosive power training. Champaign, IL: Human Kinetics

Scoles, G. 1978. Depth jumping! Does it really work? *Athletic Journal* 58(5) 48-49, 74-75.

Siff, M., and Y. Verkhoshansky. 1996. *Supertraining: Special strength training for sporting excellence.* 2d ed. Pittsburgh: Sports Support Syndicate.

Verkhoshansky, Y. 1967. Are depth jumps useful? *Track & Field* 12:9.

Verkhoshansky, Y. 1968. Are depth jumps useful? *Yessis Review of Soviet Physical Education and Sports* 3: 75-78.

Viitasalo, J.T. and Bosco, C. 1982. Electromechanical behaviour of human muscles in vertical jumps. *European Journal of Applied Physiology* 48: 253-261.

Zanon, S. 1989. Plyometrics: Past and present. *New Studies in Athletics* 4(1): 7-17.

About the Authors

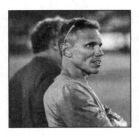

Jim Radcliffe is one of the most overlooked elements in the success of Oregon's student-athletes. Now in his third decade as the school's head strength and conditioning coach, he not only plays a significant role in the Ducks football program as the designer of the year-round conditioning calendar, but he also has been quick to aid in the athletic development of athletes in all sports in his work with Olympians and World Championship medalists.

Radcliffe has guided football, basketball, track and field, baseball, and volleyball athletes during much of his career. He furnishes the student-athletes with a variety of exercise through weight training and lifting systems and is a noted authority on exercises dealing with the improvement of speed and quickness. He became assistant strength coach at Oregon in 1985, a position he held for two years before assuming the duties of head coach in that area.

Radcliffe taught and coached a variety of sports and was the athletic trainer at Aloha High School from 1978 to 1983. He then did graduate studies at Colorado and worked in private business before joining the Ducks staff. Graduating from Pacific in Oregon with a degree in physical education and health in 1980, he played four seasons as defensive back and was captain of the special teams. Radcliffe earned his master's degree in biomechanics from Oregon.

Active in national organizations surrounding his profession, Radcliffe has been certified by USA Weightlifting, CSCCa, and the NSCA. He also has written books, been published in numerous professional journals, and produced videos on plyometrics.

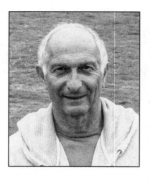

Bob Farentinos is a fitness professional and lifelong athlete. He has competed in weightlifting, cross-country skiing, and rowing and has won national titles and masters championships in all three sports. Farentinos earned his PhD in biology from the University of Colorado and spent many years as a professor and researcher at various universities, including Colorado, Michigan, Ohio State, and Johns Hopkins. He has published extensively in scientific journals and has written wildlife stories for children as well as numerous lay articles on exercise, health, and fitness.

In the 1980s, Farentinos owned and managed a sport and fitness center in Boulder, Colorado, designated as an official training facility for the U.S. ski team. At the center he trained and coached Olympic and professional athletes in cycling, running, triathlon, Nordic and alpine skiing, weightlifting, climbing, and mountaineering. During that time he also worked with athletes and coaches at the U.S. Olympic Training Center in Colorado Springs.

From 1984 through 1991, he competed in the United States Ski Association (USSA) Great American Ski Chase, a national series of 50-kilometer cross-country races, winning several age-class championships. He participated in the 1988 Winter Olympics in Calgary as a technical representative for one of his ski equipment sponsors.

Farentinos began his rowing career in 2003 at the age of 62. Within a few years he was rowing competitively, winning gold and silver medals in Northwest Regional Masters Championships in single sculling. In 2007 he won the Canadian National Masters Championship and has competed successfully since then in national and regional regattas and head races in single and double sculling.

Farentinos volunteers his time and expertise designing workout facilities and exercise programs for youth dealing with substance abuse and addiction. He uses exercise and sport to redirect their focus toward healthier and more productive lifestyles.

Farentinos lives in Portland, Oregon.

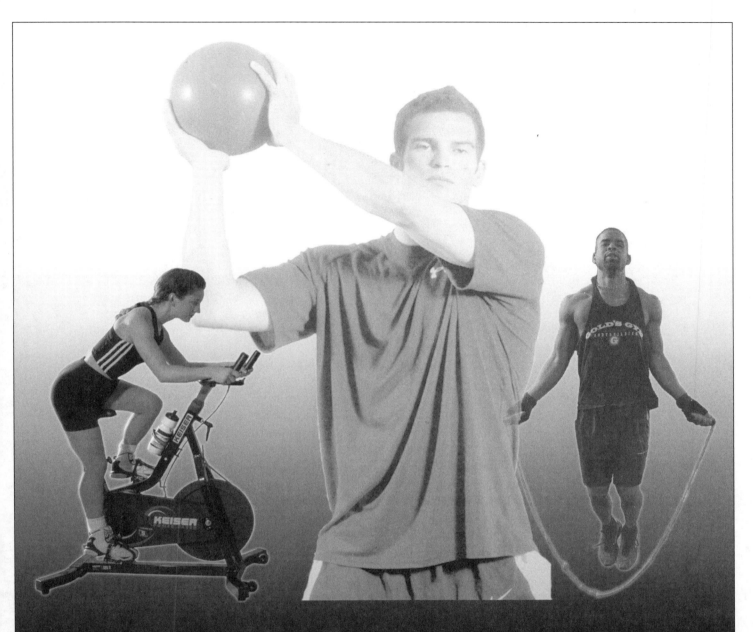

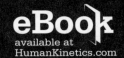